THE INSULIN RESISTANCE
DIET PLAN & COOKBOOK

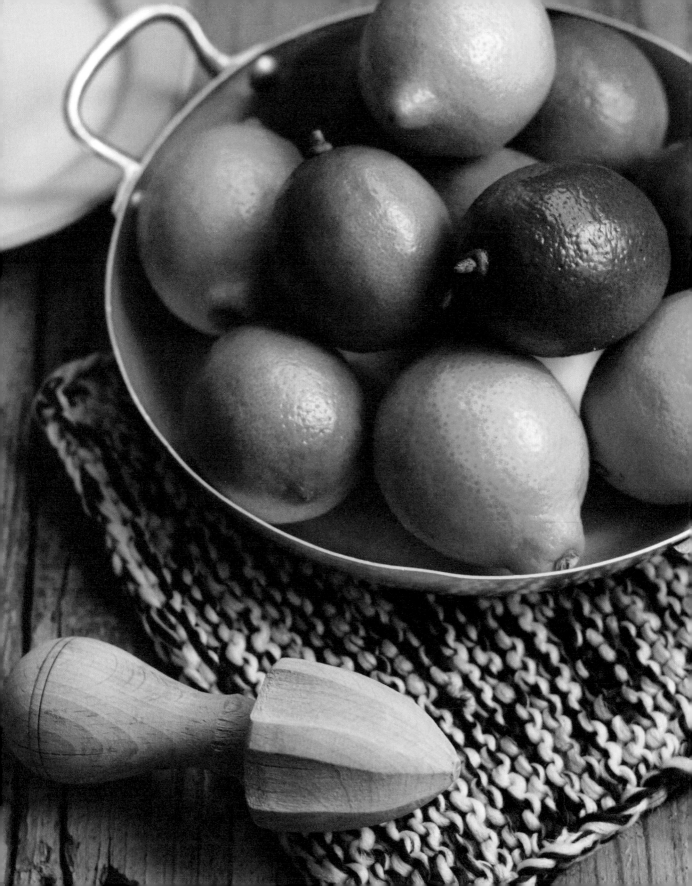

The Insulin Resistance
DIET PLAN & COOKBOOK

Lose Weight, Manage PCOS,
and Prevent Prediabetes

TARA SPENCER

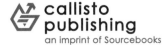
callisto
publishing
an imprint of Sourcebooks

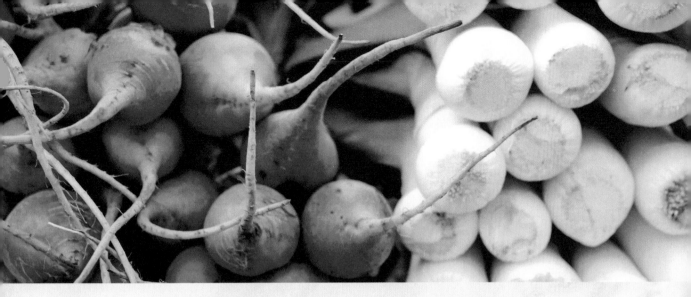

A FRESH START FOR A HEALTHIER YOU

As many as 75 percent of Americans are insulin-resistant. Most of them have no idea. But if you're reading this book, you or someone you love may have just received that diagnosis. Fortunately, learning to manage and overcome insulin resistance through mindful and healthy eating can help you reach your optimal metabolic health. Here are a few of the conditions that the Insulin Resistance Diet can improve:

Metabolic Syndrome: This condition is characterized by high blood pressure, high blood triglycerides, and low levels of "good" cholesterol (HDL)—all of which can be reversed by increasing insulin sensitivity.

Obesity: Overcoming insulin resistance and losing weight go hand in hand. Normalizing hormone production by tackling insulin resistance is a natural weight-loss method.

Polycystic Ovarian Syndrome (PCOS): While there is currently no cure for PCOS, many with this condition have discovered that overcoming insulin resistance can reverse symptoms such as irregular menstrual cycles and acne, and even help with fertility.

Prediabetes: Almost everyone who has prediabetes is insulin resistant. Following the Insulin Resistance Diet can help prevent the development of prediabetes into type 2 diabetes (and its associated risks!).

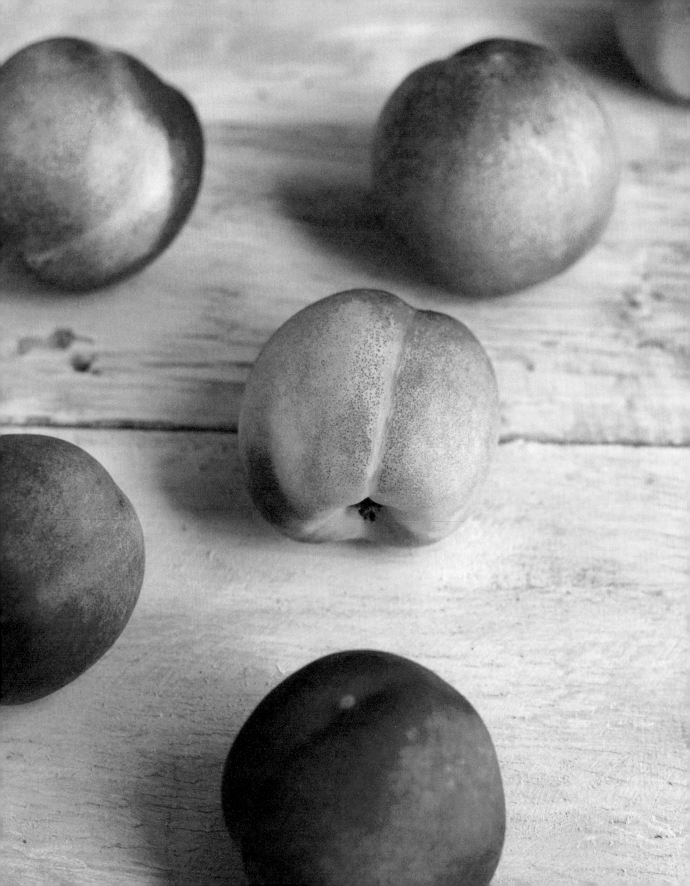

CONTENTS

FOREWORD

We've all heard the saying: "When you have your health, you have everything." Yet if you're like many people, you've tried every diet, only to gain more weight. Maybe you struggle with high blood pressure or have high cholesterol levels.

If this sounds familiar, you may suffer from insulin resistance. With this condition, excessive glucose accumulates in the bloodstream. The body then produces more insulin to stabilize blood sugar levels and stores excess glucose as fat. In more than 15 years as a registered dietitian, I've seen clients too often diet in the name of health, including skipping meals and denying hunger. This harmful behavior impacts insulin levels, blood pressure, energy levels—and self-esteem. If you've been diagnosed with insulin resistance or prediabetes, making positive changes in lifestyle, diet, and exercise can reverse its course. This doesn't mean following an over-restrictive diet or chronic dieting. When combined with high insulin levels, as in the case of PCOS (polycystic ovarian syndrome), dieting changes brain chemistry—intensifying cravings and bingeing and lowering self-esteem. Weight-cycling studies suggest that dieting actually increases inflammation and insulin levels, perpetuating the cycle.

Clients frequently come to me with tired metabolisms, insulin resistance, prediabetes, PCOS, and obesity. To help, I give them permission to trust their body and listen to its needs via signals of hunger and satiety. Together, we make small changes to food choices and meal composition, while boosting physical activity. In a study of more than 3,000 people with insulin resistance at high risk for type 2 diabetes, the Diabetes Prevention and Control Program (DPP) found that even minimal weight loss through 150 minutes of weekly physical activity and positive dietary modification lowered participants' risk of diabetes by 58 percent. I use this same curriculum with my clients. Small changes really do produce significant results. That is what this book is all about.

As Tara explains, when following this simple plan, you'll want to take the holistic approach. Eliminate processed junk, white flour–based ingredients, and foods high in saturated fats, refined sugars, and salt. Ease up on any restrictive thinking. Instead, eat regular meals and snacks, and focus on minimally processed foods. Visualize your plate: Aim to fill half with colorful, nutrient-dense, non-starchy vegetables like kale and broccoli, and antioxidant-rich fruits like berries and citrus; fill one quarter with high-fiber whole grains that lower glucose and insulin levels, like oats and barley; finally, eat one portion of lean protein. Skip fatty meats and full-fat dairy, but enjoy seeds, nuts, avocado, olives, and vegetable oils. On page 28, you'll find a handy list of foods with the most blood sugar–stabilizing effects plus those that promote fat storage.

Let's not forget that other essential component: exercise. A healthy lifestyle combines metabolism-boosting, muscle-building activities with heart-strengthening cardiovascular exercise, but the real key for improving insulin sensitivity is regular activity. Pressed for time? Tara's sample exercises and routines (see page 44) fit even the busiest schedule.

Most important, this book imparts one of the most valuable skills for achieving wellness: self-compassion. Please take heart. It's possible to alleviate your symptoms naturally, without the help of drugs. Taking charge of your lifestyle and nutrition will do wonders to restore your well-deserved good health.

—Jennifer Koslo, PhD, RDN, CSSD, LD, CPT

INTRODUCTION

If you're struggling with insulin resistance, then you're not alone. There are different reasons why people develop this condition, but the physical and emotional toll it takes is something we all share.

A few years ago, my body was a source of much unhappiness and confusion for me. I exercised daily and followed a healthy diet, but I still gained weight rapidly. I felt fat and bloated, but suffered from intense hunger and strong cravings. My energy levels rose and fell without any logical pattern, and I fainted three times within a year.

My doctors dismissed my symptoms as the ordinary hormonal fluctuations of a twenty-something-year-old woman. I blamed myself and decided I wasn't working hard enough on my fitness or being strict enough on my diet. The reality was, I was working too hard and being too restrictive.

It was not until I further researched my symptoms and sought out the expertise of a specialist that I learned I had insulin resistance, and was eventually diagnosed with polycystic ovarian syndrome (PCOS).

In my case, the two conditions were triggered by years of eating too little and exercising too much. I was living off less than 1,200 calories per day—not enough to fuel for lying in bed all day, let alone the multiple hours of exercise I had pushed myself to perform.

The result of my unhealthy dietary and exercise practice was a slowed metabolism, which created hormonal imbalances within my body. During those years, I did not have a regular menstrual cycle, and I started gaining weight, particularly around my midsection. In addition to limiting my caloric intake, I'd tried eliminating carbohydrates, but that only led to extreme cravings followed by inevitable binges and guilt.

Once I received my diagnosis, I became frustrated by my body's lack of response to traditional treatment methods. That's when I set out to manage my insulin resistance and PCOS through natural treatment methods instead.

Using my knowledge and experience as a certified nutritionist and personal trainer, I learned how to take control of my diet and exercise regime to improve and, eventually, overcome my insulin resistance. In the process, I learned to manage the symptoms of my PCOS, regained a healthy menstrual cycle, healed my metabolism, and lost the weight my body had been stubbornly retaining for years.

Dealing with these two conditions taught me to listen to my body, and through simple trial and error, determined the best way to nurture it. I learned how to treat my body with the kindness and love it deserves, and to understand the crucial role emotional health plays in overcoming a medical condition. I learned how to be patient with my body when it came to trying new foods, and to accept that significant changes would not occur overnight. I stopped fixating on the way my body looked, and instead focused on the way I felt during the recovery process: happier, more energetic, and stronger than I had felt in years.

The Insulin Resistance Diet Plan & Cookbook outlines exactly how I optimized my health by following a specific diet and modifying my exercise regime. It is for those of you who feel frustrated by traditional treatment methods, just as I did. It is also for those who seek a more natural means of improving their insulin resistance by addressing the very factor that likely led to their developing the condition in the first place: their diet.

This book provides a 28-day meal plan, and clearly defines which foods to enjoy in abundance and which to avoid. Accompanying the plan are 100 delicious, nutritious, easy-to-prepare recipes to kickstart a healthier way of living. This new lifestyle will help you overcome insulin resistance, and if applicable to you, it can help control PCOS, halt the progress of prediabetes, eliminate excess weight, and improve metabolic syndrome.

Finally, this book will teach you that achieving these outcomes is not simply a question of following the right diet or exercise regime, but rebuilding your self-confidence and healing all aspects of your internal health. With *The Insulin Resistance Diet Plan & Cookbook*, you're taking a crucial step in reclaiming your health for the rest of your life.

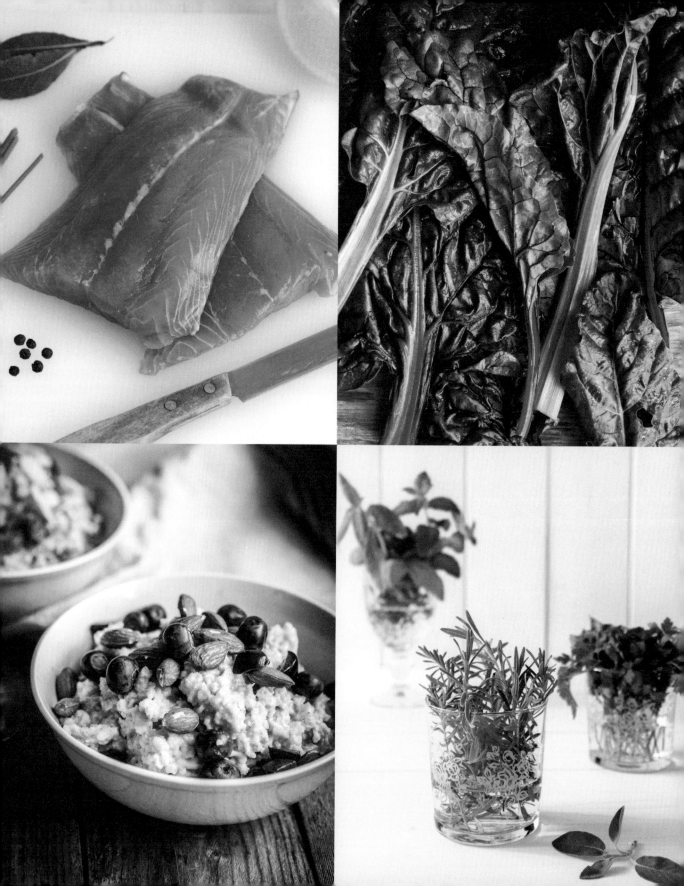

PART I

Overcoming Insulin Resistance

———

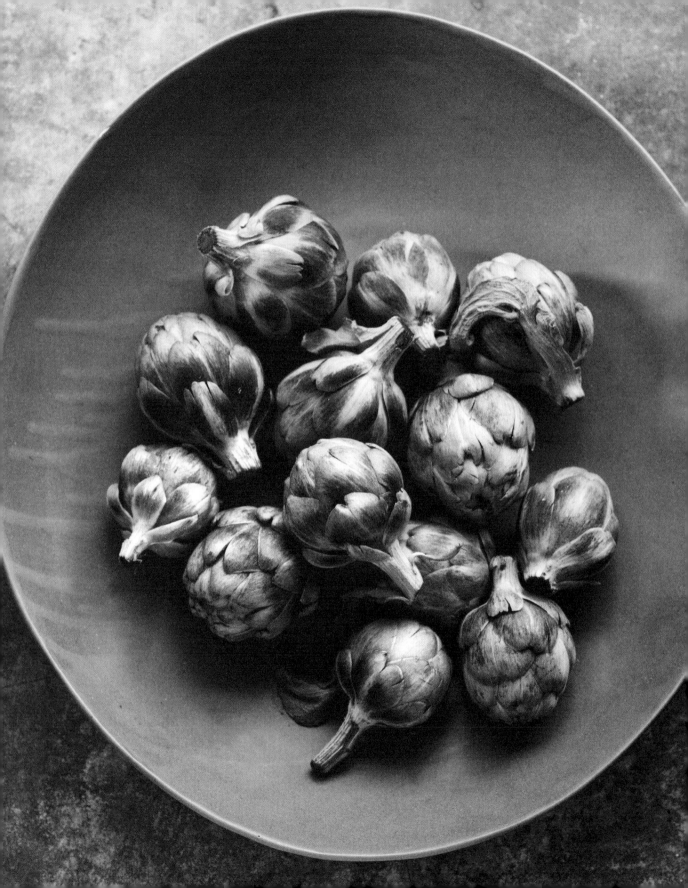

CHAPTER ONE

Understanding the Problem

Insulin resistance can be a frustrating condition. You may have cut out sugary foods and stepped up your exercise since being diagnosed, and still found that the condition won't go away. The first step to overcoming insulin resistance is to understand the connection between insulin and your metabolism. Not only is insulin needed for a healthy metabolism, but an unhealthy metabolism can lead to insulin resistance.

This chapter explains the basic relationship between food, metabolism, and insulin resistance, with brief descriptions of metabolic function, the critical role of food, and how insulin resistance manifests itself. It spells out exactly what the Insulin Resistance Diet involves, and what to expect when you begin to follow it.

A great deal of research has been conducted on the subject of insulin resistance, and if you are interested in learning more, look at the Resources section at the end of this book for a list of helpful organizations and websites.

Always consult your health care provider before making any significant changes to your diet, including the nutritional recommendations presented in the following pages. This book is a great resource, but it is no substitute for the advice of a health care practitioner.

Metabolism Basics

Your body needs energy to function. Moving, breathing, thinking, circulating blood, and growing and repairing cells are all dependent on the energy provided by the food you eat. It's your metabolism that gives your body the ability to extract that energy from food: a set of chemical reactions that both stores food molecules and converts them into energy. The metabolism is so crucial to daily function that death occurs if it shuts down. This is why your metabolism is a constant process. This process, however, does not always function efficiently.

The metabolism is often incorrectly associated with how quickly one is able to burn energy. For example, someone who remains thin no matter how much they eat tends to be credited with a fast metabolism. Conversely, some people blame their slow metabolism for gaining weight when they even look at a cupcake. What people are actually referring to here is their basal metabolic rate (BMR)—not their metabolism.

BMR is the amount of energy burned when you are at rest. In other words, your BMR is the number of calories you need to do nothing other than lie in bed all day. The average BMR in the United States is 1,493 calories for women and 1,662 calories for men (Hutchison, 2014). Your BMR is thought to account for about 70 percent of the calories you burn each day (Mayo Clinic, Sept. 2014).

It is unlikely, however, that a person's BMR—even if it is below average—is the main cause of their weight gain. Ultimately, an increase in weight results when the number of calories you consume is greater than the number you expend.

Alongside your BMR, the amount of calories you burn in a day depends on several factors:

›	**Gender:** Men almost always burn more calories than women, since their muscle-to-fat ratio is typically higher.

> **Age:** The amount of calories burned each day slows down with age due to reduced muscle mass, hormonal changes, and a decline in activity levels.

> **Genetics:** To a certain extent, genetics determines whether you have a naturally faster or slower metabolism, especially if you have any kind of genetic disorder.

> **Height and Weight:** A person with a larger build requires more calories than a person with a smaller one.

> **Body Composition:** A body with a higher percentage of muscle mass in relation to body fat will burn more calories at rest. Two people may be the exact same height and weight, but the person with more muscle will burn more calories. This is because muscle tissue requires more energy to maintain than fat tissue.

> **Activity Level:** The more active you are, the more calories you will burn.

> **Dietary Intake:** Even the act itself of digesting and absorbing food, known as thermogenesis, can burn anywhere between 100 and 800 calories per day (Mayo Clinic, Sept. 2014).

> **Environmental Factors:** Your weight can be affected by sleep, stress, and even weather conditions.

> **Hormonal Factors:** Finally, and perhaps most importantly, your hormonal state can alter your natural metabolism. Conditions such as hypothyroidism and insulin resistance tend to slow down your metabolism.

Weight gain, however, doesn't just occur from eating too much; weight gain can also occur from eating too *little*. When you severely restrict your calories, your metabolism has to slow down to adjust to that new caloric intake, and whatever incoming energy is provided tends to be stored rather than burned. The medical term for this response is *adaptive thermogenesis*. Very low calorie diets may lead to severe bingeing episodes. Over the long term, bingeing can make weight loss almost impossible.

After consuming an average of 1,200 calories a day for a period of time, I switched to eating 1,500 calories for a few consecutive days. In theory, this calorie change should have stimulated weight loss, but instead, I gained weight. I'd eaten too little for too long, causing my metabolism to slow down. The result was that my body held on to the extra energy in anticipation of being starved once again. During this time, I also struggled with bingeing on weekends, when my body fought back against an inadequate consumption of food during the week. Over time, I was able to rebuild my metabolism so that I am now able to lose weight eating approximately 2,300 calories per day, while having no issues with bingeing whatsoever.

Ideally, you should try to find the right number of calories that allows your body to receive all the nutrients it needs, while also keeping its metabolic rate high. The Insulin Resistance Diet offered in this book does not involve calorie counting, but the meal plans do contain a suitable number of calories to encourage weight loss in overweight individuals while also maintaining a healthy metabolism.

THE FUNCTION OF INSULIN

If you've been diagnosed with insulin resistance, you are probably aware that your body has an issue with insulin, but you may not know what that really means. Insulin is a hormone made by the beta cells in the pancreas, and it plays a crucial role in your metabolism. The main responsibilities of insulin are to regulate the level of glucose in your blood and enable the absorption of nutrients into your cells.

When your pancreas is healthy, it delivers small doses of insulin throughout the day and extra insulin at meal times. After you eat, your blood sugar level rises, stimulating your body to release insulin into the bloodstream. Think of insulin as a key—it "unlocks" your body's cells so they can use glucose for energy. Insulin also acts as a transporter. If your bloodstream contains more sugar than your cells need, insulin helps move the glucose to the liver, where it is stored as glycogen until needed later—such as between meals or during physical activity. The higher your blood sugar level, the more insulin the pancreas releases.

For some people, though, the body's cells build up a resistance to insulin and remain "locked." With nowhere else to go, the glucose may build up in the bloodstream, which in turn triggers the release of more insulin. The long-term repercussions of insulin resistance include the development of diabetes. When insulin levels are high, your body is not able to utilize fat as an energy source, and this can result in weight gain.

The Role of Food

What you eat is as important as the amount of calories you eat, especially when trying to overcome insulin resistance. The type of food you consume directly affects your metabolism and insulin response. Food is composed of three macronutrients: protein, carbohydrate, and fat, and each of these macronutrients affects your metabolism in a different way.

One gram of protein or carbohydrate provides four calories, while one gram of fat contains nine calories. A calorie is the base unit of heat measurement related to metabolic rate. It measures how much energy a particular food provides to the body. Of course, if you do eat more calories than your body requires, it doesn't matter whether those calories come from protein, carbohydrates, or fat—the extra fuel will be stored in the body as fat.

Eating too few calories can be equally problematic. When you do not eat enough food, your body's endocrine, immunological, and nervous systems begin to malfunction. The result is often hormonal imbalances, thyroid problems, and insulin resistance. When you are in a state of extreme caloric restriction, your body does everything possible to return to a state of *homeostasis*, or equilibrium—including slowing down your metabolic rate. A slow metabolism affects your energy levels, your digestive and hormonal health, and your ability to lose weight. In my case, severely restricting my calories increased my adrenal testosterone production and reduced my estrogen levels. Those hormonal changes severely disrupted my menstrual cycle and made losing weight extremely difficult.

Certain foods can increase your metabolic rate, either because of the specific minerals these foods contain or because of their thermogenic effect (the amount of calories burned by digesting them). Some common metabolism-boosting foods include lean meats, chile peppers, and caffeine. Conversely, other foods—such as refined carbohydrates, alcohol, foods high in saturated or hydrogenated fat, and those that contain a high amount of pesticides—can have a negative effect on your metabolism (*Prevention*, 2014). Be sure to choose the foods that contribute to a healthy diet during your quest to build a healthy metabolism.

PROTEIN

Protein is responsible for the growth and repair of body tissue. When glycogen stores are low, protein is also used as an energy source. There are two types of protein: complete and incomplete. Complete proteins contain all nine essential amino acids, and include foods such as meat, fish, poultry, eggs, soy, and dairy products. Incomplete proteins are foods such as cereals, legumes, fruits, and vegetables.

Protein has a high thermogenic effect. It is estimated that 25 to 30 percent of the calories in protein are expended, or burned up, as food is digested. The corresponding figures for carbohydrate (6 to 8 percent) and fat (2 to 3 percent) are much lower (Gunnars, 2013). This means that if you were to consume 100 calories of protein, the process of digestion would burn 25 to 30 calories, and your body would only have 70 to 75 calories available to use after digestion. Conversely, if you were to consume 100 calories of fat, your body would have 97 to 98 calories to use.

CARBOHYDRATE

Carbohydrates are your body's preferred source of energy. In the American diet, carbohydrates typically account for the majority of calories. Carbohydrates provide energy for your everyday life and exercise. They can help with cravings, improve sleep quality, and even assist with fat loss. If you have insulin resistance, however, your body has a poor tolerance for carbohydrates because, unlike fat or protein, the macronutrient is broken down into glucose. Even so, carbohydrates still play an important role in the Insulin Resistance Diet and should not be eliminated completely—especially if you hope to regain a normal insulin response in the future.

There are two types of carbohydrates: simple and complex. Simple carbohydrates, or sugars, are quick-digesting sources of energy, but they also cause sudden surges and drops in blood sugar levels and should be avoided by people with insulin resistance. Simple carbohydrates include foods such as fruit, chocolate, crackers, and white flour–based products like bread and pasta.

Complex carbohydrates, or starches, provide a gradual release of energy, as well as valuable vitamins and minerals. They are a much better choice for insulin-resistant individuals. Complex carbohydrates include foods such as potatoes, beans, oatmeal, whole-grain flours, whole wheat, and products made from whole grains.

FAT

Fat isn't something to be avoided. It is an essential nutrient that protects organs, regulates body temperature, processes vitamins, and repairs body tissue. Contrary to popular belief, consuming fat will not make you fat—provided you eat the right type.

There are several types of fat. Monounsaturated fats improve blood cholesterol levels and improve insulin sensitivity. This type of fat is found in olives, beef, nuts, seeds, and avocados. Polyunsaturated fats—found in oily fish, nuts, and seeds—are another "good" fat. They improve blood cholesterol levels and may reduce the risk for type 2 diabetes.

Saturated fat has been linked to an increased risk of heart disease and type 2 diabetes. It mainly comes from animal sources of food, such as red meat, poultry, and full-fat dairy. There is much debate in the health community as to what extent certain saturated fats can be beneficial to health, especially coconut oil. However, this diet recommends the elimination of saturated fat to the greatest extent possible.

Trans fat is made from hydrogenated oil and is linked to cardiovascular disease. It is commonly found in processed foods, especially processed snack foods such as chips and crackers, and packaged sweets like cookies and cakes (Mayo Clinic, Aug. 2014).

Developing Insulin Resistance

What is insulin resistance? Simply put, the condition exists when your body's cells have grown resistant to the effects of insulin. This means that glucose cannot enter the cells and instead remains in the bloodstream, causing high blood sugar levels. To properly utilize carbohydrates, the body needs to produce greater amounts of insulin. But since the bloodstream is already circulating more than enough insulin, this encourages the body to store the glucose as fat.

One of the biggest problems of insulin resistance is that it often has no symptoms. In fact, people often remain undiagnosed until the condition leads to the development of type 2 diabetes. Occasionally, you may experience symptoms such as concentration difficulties, depression, increased blood pressure, intense hunger, intestinal bloating, or lethargy. You may also suffer from strong cravings for sweet and salty food. You may also have experienced weight gain or have had difficulty losing weight. I personally suffered for years from bloating that wasn't caused by food allergies. I also experienced strong cravings every day due to the added effect of undereating. Both of these symptoms affected my self-confidence and led to feelings of depression. If you suspect you may be insulin resistant, determine how many of the risk factors you have in the following section, and then take a blood test to check your blood sugar level.

Diabetic Care Services estimates that as many as 75 percent of Americans suffer some degree of insulin resistance, and most are unaware of it. The condition is largely caused by following a diet high in refined carbohydrates while leading a sedentary lifestyle. Excessive amounts of insulin are released to process the high levels of glucose that accompany the average American diet. Over time, this constant production of insulin causes the beta cells of the pancreas to malfunction, which, in turn, results in the eventual intolerance to carbohydrates, and consequent insulin resistance.

Crash diets can also create insulin resistance, especially a diet that restricts carbohydrate intake over a prolonged period of time. A 2010 study (Jornayvaz et al.) debunked the myth that only high-carbohydrate diets cause insulin resistance. The study showed that low-carbohydrate, high-fat, ketogenic diets are equally problematic when it comes to lowering insulin receptor sensitivity—even if the diets do not cause weight gain. Without carbohydrates to regularly stimulate the release of insulin, the beta cells in your pancreas become damaged. At some point, you will consume some form of carbohydrate, and your body will simply not know how to cope.

Chronic dieters tend to gain fat much more easily than those who have never dieted at all. When you follow a low-carbohydrate diet for an extended period, your fat cells have a heightened level of insulin sensitivity. This is one reason why 95 percent of crash dieters regain the weight they lost (O'Meara, 2015).

When people revert from a highly processed, high-carbohydrate diet to a restrictive, low-carbohydrate diet, their bodies continue to secrete insulin, despite the lack of carbohydrates in their systems. This can lead to all kinds of hormonal problems, weight gain, and an eventual slowdown of insulin production.

When insufficient quantities of insulin are released, a variety of serious health conditions can result—including diabetes. There are two types of diabetes. Type 1 occurs when the beta cells produce either no insulin at all or a very limited amount. Type 2 occurs when the beta cells have an impaired ability to manufacture insulin, or when the insulin receptors on individual cells become insensitive and stop responding to the existing insulin in the bloodstream (*You and Your Hormones*, 2015).

It's clear that insulin resistance cannot be managed simply by following a restrictive diet. The correct way to overcome the condition is by eating whole, unprocessed foods and teaching your body to efficiently process carbohydrates once again. These are principles of the Insulin Resistance Diet.

RISK FACTORS FOR DEVELOPING INSULIN RESISTANCE

Certain factors can increase your chances of developing insulin resistance. Some of them are within your control, while others are not. The good news is that the two biggest contributors to insulin resistance are within your power to manage. These are—according to the National Institute of Diabetes and Digestive and Kidney Diseases (NIDDKD)—physical inactivity and carrying excess amounts of weight.

Controllable Factors

When it comes to developing insulin resistance, you can take charge of the following factors.

PHYSICAL INACTIVITY: When you regularly partake in exercise, your muscles burn their glucose stores for energy and subsequently refill their reserves with glucose in the bloodstream, without the direct need for insulin. This helps naturally keep blood glucose levels in balance. Furthermore, your muscles are more sensitive to insulin after exercise, which helps reverse insulin resistance. When you do not exercise regularly, your blood sugar levels remain high, and you are more likely to become overweight.

EXCESS WEIGHT: Being overweight or obese is a primary factor for developing insulin resistance. Excess body fat, particularly around the waist, can affect natural hormone levels. This change can cause cardiovascular disease, cholesterol problems, high blood pressure, and insulin resistance (NIDDKD, 2014). Losing weight by following a healthy diet and exercising regularly can help improve insulin resistance and reduce the risk of developing type 2 diabetes.

EATING TOO MUCH SUGAR: Eating foods that contain high amounts of sugar disrupts your endocrine system. Sugar tricks the body into releasing insulin at the wrong time or in the wrong quantities.

EATING TOO MUCH FAT: Diets high in saturated and trans fats are closely linked to the development of insulin resistance. One study demonstrated that rats developed insulin resistance after just three weeks of following a high-fat diet (Kraegen et al., 1991).

STEROID USE: Steroids affect the body's natural insulin response. The elevated quantity of sex hormones—particularly testosterone—in steroids inhibits insulin signaling, which can lead to insulin resistance.

CIGARETTE SMOKING: Nicotine impairs the action of insulin, slowing down the normal rate of glucose disposal (Targher et al., 1997).

DIFFICULTY SLEEPING: Sleep issues—particularly sleep apnea—are highly associated with an increased risk of insulin resistance, obesity, and type 2 diabetes (NIDDKD, 2014).

Uncontrollable Factors

The following factors, unfortunately, are beyond your control when it comes to developing insulin resistance.

GENETIC PREDISPOSITION: A family history of type 2 diabetes will increase your chance of becoming insulin resistant. If your genetic background is African, Alaskan, Asian, Hispanic/Latino, Pacific Islander, First Nations, or any indigenous peoples of the Americas, the risk is believed to be higher.

AGE: Being 40 years of age or older will increase your risk of developing insulin resistance.

GIVING BIRTH TO A BABY WEIGHING MORE THAN NINE POUNDS: A baby's size at birth is a reflection of its intrauterine environment. Large babies and their mothers are both at a higher risk of developing insulin resistance and type 2 diabetes (Yajnik et al., 2003). Women who are overweight or obese during pregnancy are more likely to give birth to heavier babies, so weight management is one controllable aspect of this factor.

HAVING POLYCYSTIC OVARIAN SYNDROME (PCOS): Just as steroid users have a greater risk of developing insulin resistance due to their body's higher level of sex hormones, so do women with PCOS. Symptoms of PCOS include cysts on the ovaries, irregular or absent menstrual cycles, and elevated sex hormones— the last of which causes acne, facial hair, and excess weight gain. PCOS is very common—about 10 percent of the western female population suffer from it

WHO IS MOST AT RISK FOR INSULIN RESISTANCE?

A number of controllable and uncontrollable factors determine one's likelihood of developing insulin resistance. The probability is especially high for individuals with these conditions:

> **PCOS:** The syndrome is linked with excess androgen production, a hormone that acts directly on peripheral tissues to promote insulin resistance. At least 50 percent of women with PCOS are insulin resistant, and around 10 percent of all insulin-resistant women suffer from PCOS (Dunaif, 1997). Staggeringly, about 80 percent of obese women with PCOS will develop insulin resistance by the age of 40 (*Healthy Women*, 2012).

> **Prediabetes:** According to the National Institute of Diabetes and Digestive and Kidney Diseases (NIDDKD), almost everyone who is prediabetic is insulin resistant. With prediabetes, blood glucose levels are higher than normal, but not high enough to warrant a diagnosis of diabetes. The US Department of Health and Human Services estimated that at least 86 million American adults aged 20 or older had prediabetes in 2012. The NIDDKD forecasts that prediabetic persons will have type 2 diabetes within 10 years unless they change their lifestyle.

> **Metabolic syndrome:** This condition shares many of the same characteristics as prediabetes. Most who suffer from it are also insulin resistant, so the two terms are often used interchangeably. According to Alberti et al. (2009), you have metabolic syndrome if three or more of the following symptoms are present: a large waist size (40 inches or more for men, 35 inches or more for women); high blood pressure (130/85 or above); high blood triglycerides (150 milligrams per deciliter or above); elevated fasting plasma glucose levels (100 milligrams per deciliter or above); and low high-density lipoprotein cholesterol levels (below 40 milligrams per deciliter in men, below 50 milligrams per deciliter in women).

> **Obesity:** Excess body fat disrupts normal hormone production. A vicious cycle develops whereby the more obese you are, the more insulin resistant you become, because the excess fat spikes cortisol—a hormone that prevents insulin from performing properly.

(Dunaif, 1997). Although PCOS can never be cured, the symptoms can be managed—primarily through dietary changes—to minimize or even reverse a state of insulin resistance.

The Insulin Resistance Diet

The good news is that insulin resistance can be treated. There are two ways to manage your insulin resistance. The first is to reduce your need for insulin by modifying your diet. The second is to increase your cells' sensitivity to insulin with regular exercise. In fact, a study showed that diet and exercise were found to be nearly twice as effective as metformin (a common drug prescribed to treat type 2 diabetes and PCOS) when it comes to preventing the onset of type 2 diabetes in individuals with insulin resistance (Knowler et al., 2002).

The ideal diet for someone suffering from insulin resistance is based on whole foods, with large quantities of protein, fiber, fruits, and vegetables. Most important, this diet should be low in sugars and white flours, with a low glycemic load. This style of eating is simpler, and more natural for most people to process and digest.

The glycemic index (GI) is a number associated with how a certain food affects a person's blood glucose level. Carbohydrates are given a glycemic number between 0 and 100, with 100 being equivalent to pure glucose. For example, if you eat a baked potato (glycemic index 85), your body's blood glucose response will be almost three times as much as it would to the same quantity of carbohydrates in black beans (glycemic index 30). (In Appendix A we've included a handy list of the glycemic index and glycemic load of many common carbohydrates.)

Fortunately, understanding the GI is fairly simple: Low-glycemic foods have a rating of 55 or less, while foods with a rating of 70 to 100 are considered to be high-GI. Medium-level foods have a glycemic index of 56 to 69. In general, people should avoid foods with a high GI, and especially if you have insulin resistance. High-glycemic carbohydrates increase your blood glucose level more rapidly, and consequently stimulate the secretion of a greater amount of insulin than foods lower on the GI. This causes your blood pressure to rise, which can lead to headaches, energy slumps, and mood swings. The consumption of low-glycemic foods, on the other hand, is less likely to cause insulin resistance and obesity due to their slower and milder effect on blood sugar (McMillan-Price and Brand-Miller, 2006).

Common high-glycemic foods include unrefined sugars (such as fruit juice, syrup, and table sugar), white bread, and unrefined corn and potato products (such as bagels, doughnuts, and white potatoes).

Low-glycemic carbohydrates include those with a higher fiber content (such as whole-grain breads, legumes, and brown rice), and non-starchy vegetables (such as asparagus, broccoli, and green beans).

The glycemic load (GL) of a food is different from its glycemic index. The GL refers to how many carbohydrates per serving the food contains. A GL of less than 10 is considered low and between 10 and 20 is considered moderate. Anything above 20 is considered high and should be avoided due to its negative impact on blood sugar. As a general rule, it is more beneficial to pay attention to a food's glycemic load than to its glycemic index. This is because some foods, such as watermelon and carrots, have a high glycemic index but would need to be consumed in enormous quantities to carry a high glycemic load.

All the carbohydrates in the Foods to Enjoy list on page 28 have a low glycemic load. These foods, combined with foods containing high levels of protein and healthy unsaturated fats, make the Insulin Resistance Diet anti-inflammatory, high in antioxidants, metabolism-boosting, and ideal for balancing your blood sugar levels.

GUIDELINES FOR THE INSULIN RESISTANCE DIET

The following are some important guidelines to keep in mind while following the Insulin Resistance Diet.

EVERY MEAL SHOULD CONTAIN A SOURCE OF PROTEIN. High-protein foods do not affect insulin levels, and are therefore the ideal choice on which to base your diet. Recommended sources of protein include lean meats, fish, poultry, eggs, and legumes.

EVERY MEAL SHOULD ALSO CONTAIN AT LEAST ONE SERVING OF VEGETABLES FROM THE APPROVED LIST. Vegetables are low in both calories and carbohydrates, making them ideal for those trying to manage their blood sugar levels. Fresh vegetables are preferable to vegetable juices, which do not contain fiber and are consequently not as filling. Raw or lightly cooked vegetables are best.

FOODS TO ENJOY AND FOODS TO AVOID

FOODS TO ENJOY

Fish (cod, halibut, herring, salmon, sardines)

Lean meats (beef, chicken, lamb, pork, turkey)

Eggs

Legumes (black beans, chickpeas, lentils, soybeans)

Low-GI vegetables (asparagus, broccoli, Brussels sprouts, cabbage, kale, spinach)

Low-GI fruits (apples, berries, cherries, peaches, pears, plums, rhubarb)

Medium-GI fruits (cantaloupes, grapes, kiwifruit)

Whole grains (amaranth, buckwheat, millet, quinoa, teff)

Extra-virgin olive oil, coconut oil, flaxseed oil

Nuts and seeds (almonds, flaxseed, macadamia nuts, pumpkin seeds, walnuts)

Garlic

Dairy alternatives (almond, coconut, hazelnut, and soy milk)

Dark chocolate

FOODS TO AVOID

Alcohol

All foods containing white sugar and flour (bagels, breads, cereals, pasta, pastries)

All foods containing high-fructose corn syrup (breakfast cereals, juices, ketchup, salad dressings, soda)

All foods containing hydrogenated oils (cakes, candy, chips, doughnuts)

Artificial sweeteners (acesulfame K, aspartame, saccharin, sorbitol)

Fish containing mercury (shark, swordfish, tuna, tilefish)

High-GI vegetables (corn, rutabagas, parsnips, potatoes, turnips)

Most dairy

Processed fruit juices

Processed oils (canola, corn, peanut, safflower, sunflower)

Red meat (unless organic or grass-fed) and organ meats

EAT ONE TO TWO SERVINGS OF FRUIT PER DAY FROM THE APPROVED LIST. Again, choose fresh fruit rather than juices for more fiber, vitamins, and minerals.

EAT REGULARLY, EVERY TWO TO FOUR HOURS. Ideally, this will mean three meals and two to three snacks per day to prevent your blood sugar levels from dropping and allow for the stable release of insulin.

CONTROL YOUR CARBOHYDRATE INTAKE. Standard dietary recommendations suggest that carbohydrates should make up as much as 65 percent of your diet (Trumbo et al., 2002). In reality, this amount is far too high for the average person, especially for someone with insulin resistance. Reducing your carbohydrate intake to a low to moderate level will improve your symptoms tremendously. Remember, it is important not to remove carbohydrates from the diet completely, since this can create problems in itself. In my own case, a low-carbohydrate diet was largely what led to my hormonal and energy problems—and did not inspire any weight loss. Although a study by Lee and Fujioka (2011) suggested that a low-carbohydrate diet is more effective than a low-fat diet to treat insulin resistance, their definition of "low-carbohydrate" meant 40 percent of your overall caloric intake—a perfectly appropriate target level for most people.

FOCUS ON THE OVERALL GL OF YOUR MEALS AS A WHOLE, RATHER THAN THE GI OF INDIVIDUAL FOODS. Never eat carbohydrates on their own. Instead, combine them with proteins and fats to slow their release into the bloodstream. For example, instead of eating just a piece of fruit or a plain baked potato, try accompanying the fruit with some yogurt or nuts, and the potato with a portion of meat.

AVOID ARTIFICIAL SWEETENERS. Although they do not contain sugar and therefore do not increase blood glucose levels, artificial sweeteners still stimulate the release of insulin. Consuming foods with artificial sweeteners also continues to fuel your desire for sweet foods, which will make cutting these foods out of your diet even more difficult.

EAT THE RIGHT KINDS OF FATS. While unsaturated fats should be an important part of your diet, be careful not to increase inflammation by consuming too many omega-6 fats, such as nuts and seeds. Instead, eat plenty of omega-3 fats in seafood. Saturated and trans fats should be avoided altogether.

CHOOSE ORGANIC PRODUCE AND ANIMAL PRODUCTS WHEREVER POSSIBLE. Meat from grain-fed animals contains more saturated fats and omega-6 oils than meat from wild or free-range animals, which also include more omega-3s.

Some good options are wild fish, free-range chicken and turkey, wild game, and grass-fed beef, buffalo, lamb, and pork.

CONSUME 30 TO 35 GRAMS OF FIBER PER DAY. A high-fiber diet helps stabilize blood sugar. Fiber not only supports a healthy digestive tract but also slows the body's absorption of carbohydrates.

LIMIT YOUR INTAKE OF DAIRY. Because consuming saturated fats can increase insulin resistance, avoid full-fat dairy.

DRINK WATER AND NONCAFFEINATED HERBAL TEAS. Caffeine has been shown to increase insulin resistance by about 15 percent (Biaggioni and Davis, 2002). You'll have more success overcoming insulin resistance if you cut out caffeine while following this diet.

Managing Expectations

Overcoming your insulin resistance doesn't happen overnight. There will be, however, both short- and long-term effects when you begin the Insulin Resistance Diet.

The long-term effects are overwhelmingly positive. Some of the short-term effects may be unpleasant. The presence of an unpleasant symptom, as well as its severity, depends on the current state of your diet. If your diet consists primarily of processed foods and few vegetables, your body will receive somewhat of a shock when switching to a more natural, whole foods-based diet.

In the short term, you may experience strong cravings, a drop in energy levels, and headaches as you "withdraw" from certain foods. This is perfectly normal and, thankfully, only temporary.

The good news is that, over the long term, you can expect to see a boost in your immune system, better digestion, an improvement in concentration levels and mood, increased energy levels, a reduction in cravings and overall hunger, reduced blood pressure, and weight loss.

I struggled with headaches and sweet cravings when I initially modified my diet, so I relied on headache medicine to assist with the withdrawal period and chewed fresh mint to help with my cravings for sweets. I felt markedly better within a few short weeks, which made dealing with a few days of discomfort completely worth the long-term benefits.

SHORT-TERM SIDE EFFECTS

Your body may have become very used to foods that are high in sugar, hydrogenated oils, or caffeine, and is likely to let you know how it feels when you deprive it of them. The following side effects are normal and may occur immediately, or after a week or two of following the Insulin Resistance Diet. Within a few weeks, though, the symptoms will become a distant memory and your body will adjust to the new diet and start experiencing the positive, longer-term effects.

Cravings

Many of the foods you will cut out have addictive properties. This means that your body will beg you to consume foods you should not be eating—such as alcohol, chips, coffee, and pastries—through strong cravings. When you tell your body that it can no longer have a certain food, it is amazing how much it will suddenly want that food. Keep healthy snacks on hand for those moments when cravings strike.

Remind yourself that this phase is only temporary and, after a few days (once the foods have been completely removed from your bloodstream), the cravings will disappear. In fact, foods that you previously enjoyed will likely taste too sweet or salty.

Headaches

Due to the addictive properties of processed foods, you may experience headaches during the first few days of the diet. You are also likely to suffer caffeine withdrawal headaches if you previously consumed a lot of caffeine. It is particularly important to ride this phase out, and have confidence that it will be over within a matter of days. This can be one of the toughest phases to get through if you are not well prepared—I stocked up on headache medicine and tried to avoid stressful, loud situations during this phase.

Reduced Energy Levels

One final uncomfortable effect you may experience during withdrawal is a reduction in energy level. As your body detoxes from high-calorie processed foods, it is common to feel lethargic. Again, the good news is that this phase is only temporary, and you will eventually end up with more energy than ever before.

LONG-TERM SIDE EFFECTS

Now that you understand some of the unfortunate side effects you may experience in the short term, let us consider some of the positive, longer-term effects of reversing insulin resistance.

Better Digestion

Many of the foods you will eliminate in this diet contain gluten, dairy, and sugar. You may be sensitive to some of these ingredients without realizing it. By minimizing your intake of these foods, you may be surprised to see an improvement in your digestive system. These improvements include a reduction in bloating, constipation, and/or diarrhea. Due to the increased intake of fiber, you will also experience more regular bowel movements.

Boosted Immune System

By eliminating highly inflammatory and potentially allergenic foods, you will improve your overall health. One of the first places this change in health will manifest is in your immune system: You will get sick less often.

Improved Concentration and Mood

When you consume high-carbohydrate and high-fat foods, you are likely to experience a sudden boost in productivity, followed by a down period. During the down period, you may find it difficult to concentrate and even feel more irritable until you get your next hit of sugar.

When you eat foods that keep your blood sugar level steady, however, those wild fluctuations in your mood go away, and you'll find it easier to concentrate for long periods of time. A wholesome diet composed of natural foods has even been shown to alleviate symptoms of depression (Sanchez-Villegas and Martinez-Gonzales, 2013).

Increased Energy Levels

Eliminating high-GI foods and drinks that provide sudden bursts of energy will teach your body to maximize its natural energy levels instead. And since you will no longer experience any significant surges or drops in your blood glucose, your energy levels will remain constant throughout the day, and the quality of your sleep will improve as well.

Reduced Blood Pressure

Following a nutritious diet that is low in sugar as well as in saturated and trans fat will help reduce your blood pressure and, in turn, decrease your risk of heart attack, heart disease, stroke, and other diseases (American Heart Association, 2015).

Reduced Cravings and Hunger

Although cutting out processed foods may initially cause an increase in cravings for sweet and salty foods, this response will lessen over time. Soon, your body will crave the natural, nurturing qualities of wholesome foods.

Keeping your blood sugar level stable throughout the day will also positively affect your hunger levels. The approved foods in this diet will release energy slowly and evenly into your bloodstream, so hunger will develop naturally and gradually.

Weight Loss

It's worth stating again that one of the best ways to control your insulin resistance is by losing weight. By going on the Insulin Resistance Diet—especially if you combine it with the recommended exercise regime in chapter 2—you will almost effortlessly see the pounds melt away. You will naturally eat fewer calories and no longer crave the foods that encourage fat storage in an insulin-resistant individual.

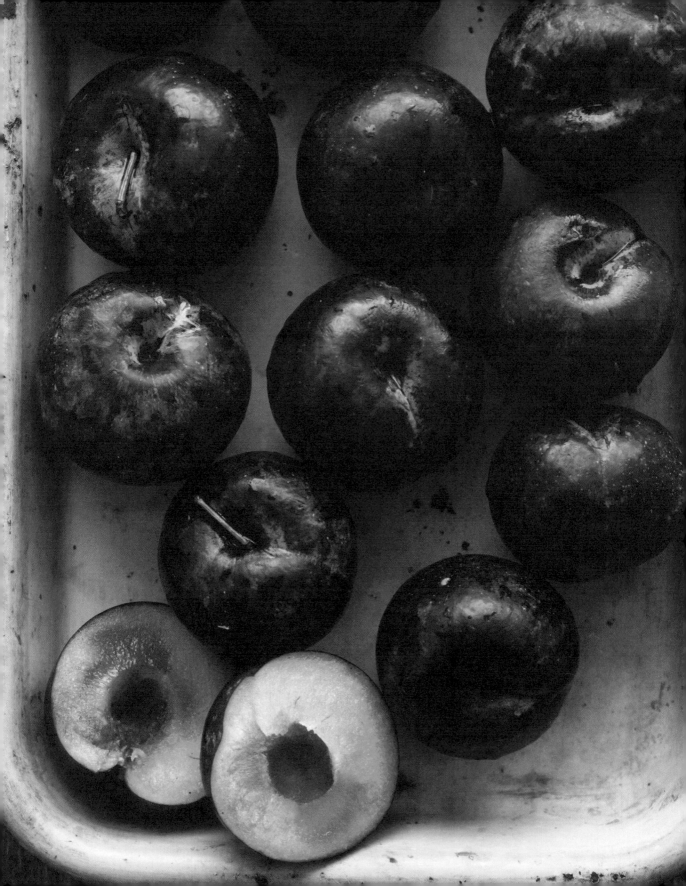

CHAPTER TWO

Intuitive Eating— and Living— for Good Health

There is an emotional aspect to nearly every recovery process, and overcoming your insulin resistance is no different. As you learn to develop and to listen to your intuition, you will come to make food choices that are right for you. Practicing self-compassion will help you avoid sabotaging yourself as you move forward toward health. This chapter also outlines the second critical factor in improving insulin resistance: Exercise.

Listening to Your Intuition

Intuition is that voice inside you that tells you what to do, even if what it's saying sometimes goes against your conscious reasoning. A significant, yet vastly underestimated aspect of overcoming any health condition is learning to listen to and trust that voice. You can certainly tell a person that a diet will cure them of an ailment and hope they will follow it. But unless that diet feels right to that person—unless they feel better for having started it and can see an improvement in their medical condition—they are unlikely to stick with it.

No one will stand by your side 24 hours a day to talk you out of those cakes, chips, and sugary drinks. And no one is watching if you slip up. The Insulin Resistance Diet relies on healthy and delicious recipes, but you must have a good reason for following the diet, and for staying on it. Allow your intuition to remind you of that reason every so often. Staying on track can be tough. Remember to keep that inner voice by your side as your cheerleader and source of constant support. This book gives you the tools to overcome your insulin resistance, but you need the right frame of mind to make it a success.

Don't expect absolute perfection from yourself. You may find the journey toward recovery or management of your condition too challenging at times, and it is completely normal to slip up on occasion. Becoming in tune with your intuition takes time. Remember that you are not alone in this process, and almost everyone will stumble at some point. During particularly challenging times, I reminded myself to focus on making small amounts of progress each day, rather than allowing one off-track day to derail my entire journey.

Once you get started, focus on the benefits—like increased energy levels, reduced mood fluctuations, and improved digestion. Remind yourself that you are taking positive steps to improve your health, and no dessert in the world is sweet enough to risk compromising that. Ask yourself if giving in to a momentary craving is worth sacrificing your ultimate goal. Your intuition may remind you how bad—both physically and emotionally—you might feel after eating inappropriate foods.

Of course, you cannot expect to follow the diet perfectly for the rest of your life! Try to limit your intake of the Foods to Avoid listed in chapter 1, but don't be afraid of occasionally doing what is best for your body in the moment. Rather than viewing a special piece of birthday cake or a restaurant meal with your family as cheating, accept the treat as a normal part of life. If your intuition tells you to enjoy a high-carbohydrate meal lovingly prepared by your children just this once, listen to it.

The trick is to learn how to get right back on track without letting one off-plan meal completely unravel your progress. You might even be surprised to find that your intuition will tell you to decline whatever high-carbohydrate or high-fat treat is dangling in front of your nose, and opt instead for a nourishing meat and vegetable dish packed full of nutrients.

PRACTICING SELF-COMPASSION

Self-compassion is an essential tool in helping you maintain healthy habits. Expressing sympathy and concern toward your own failures, inadequacies, and sufferings will keep you moving forward toward a healthier life. Dr. Kristin Neff, a pioneer in scientific research on self-compassion, specifies common humanity, mindfulness, and self-kindness as the three key aspects of self-compassion. (See the Resources section for more information.)

When you begin your journey toward repairing insulin resistance, ask if you are treating yourself with the same kindness, patience, and compassion you would extend to a loved one during a time of suffering. If you had a friend who embraced a new lifestyle to take charge of her health, would you fill them with feelings of shame and body hatred (see Shame and Body Image, page 39), or would you be proud and offer encouragement?

If you stumble on your diet or temporarily leave it all together, treat yourself with kindness. I initially felt terribly guilty when I had to eat non-optimal foods at a work function or a family dinner. I would beat myself up, worrying that a single meal had reversed all the good progress I'd made up to that point. I soon learned that this was a ridiculous mind-set: Just as one healthy meal will not reverse your insulin resistance, one unhealthy meal will not trigger diabetes. I was by no means perfect in my food choices. By keeping focused on the long-term picture, though, I was able to make decisions that led me in the right direction and, ultimately, to my goal.

Accept that mistakes happen, remind yourself that nobody is perfect, and understand that it's only human to sometimes fall short of ideals. Do not feel guilty; just get right back on task. Shift your mind-set away from wanting to change yourself because you believe you are worthless or unacceptable in your current state; instead, seek changes to make yourself healthier or happier.

Tips for Practicing Self-Compassion

Whenever you feel any type of suffering—whether that be anger, shame, guilt, or even boredom—take it as a sign that you need to take time for self-compassion. Set aside 10 minutes to engage in any of the following activities.

REVISE YOUR LANGUAGE: Consider the way you talk to yourself. Are you kind and forgiving, or harsh and overly critical? For example, don't tell yourself you are a failure for eating food on the prohibited list. You don't have to tell yourself to give up. Remind yourself that you are human, and eating one "wrong" thing will not entirely derail your progress.

JOURNAL: Many people benefit from taking a moment to write down their thoughts. Journaling can help you process the difficult events of your day, and help you avoid repeating such experiences in the future.

REPEAT A POSITIVE AFFIRMATION: When you are struggling, try speaking aloud. Try saying one of these phrases: "This is only a temporary moment of suffering," "Suffering is a normal aspect of life," "I am not alone," or "I must be kind to myself during this difficult time."

TAKE PART IN A RELAXING ACTIVITY: Do something you enjoy, something that will also decrease your stress level. Try reading, going for a walk, listening to music, or—my personal favorite—taking a bubble bath.

GIVE YOURSELF A SELF-COMPASSION BREAK: Close your eyes and notice what you're feeling. Try to name the emotion by saying to yourself, "This is anger," or "I'm feeling sad." Then, remind yourself that you're not alone in feeling this way—many people in the world feel this way, too. Finally, place your hands on your belly, over your heart, or on your cheek and say, "May I treat myself with kindness."

PRACTICE MEDITATION: Meditation will help you retrain your brain so that positive statements of self-compassion become more natural. Dr. Neff offers a number of self-guided meditations on her website. (See Resources.)

SHAME AND BODY IMAGE

When you first begin your journey to overcome insulin resistance, it is common to have a poor body image. You may feel a sense of shame that your body progressed to its current condition, or that you didn't take steps to reverse the damage sooner. But it is important to put down the self-blame and realize that this is simply a condition, one that you can overcome. And it starts by not shaming your own body.

I used to struggle with poor body image and body dysmorphia, a disorder in which a person focuses excessively on perceived flaws in their appearance. Changes in my perception of my body occurred when I began to focus on my improvements in health and athleticism instead of my physical appearance. Over time, this made me feel much more confident—and my positive internal feelings translated into a positive external appearance.

Take a moment to acknowledge and accept any negative feelings you may have about yourself, and then do your best to let them go. Remind yourself that the hardest part is over; you have recognized the factors contributing to your insulin resistance and committed to a plan to heal your health. There is no shame in that. In fact, you can feel proud.

Be kind to yourself, and remember, you are not alone. Millions of people are in the same situation. Rather than dwelling on your negative symptoms, focus on the shorter-term benefits of the Insulin Resistance Diet, such as increased energy levels and improved moods. If you are feeling even a little bit better, hold onto those moments of recognition and remember them on hard days.

During this time of healing, I recommend removing toxic and negative elements from your environment. This may involve avoiding (or ignoring) magazines, television programs, and advertisements that depict a narrow view of what bodies should look like—usually one that idolizes a thin female figure and a muscular male body. Instead, find body-positive media that encourages you to accept your body as beautiful—and dismiss mainstream "beauty standards."

In addition, consider disconnecting yourself from people in your life that judge you based on your appearance, or who only want to talk about their bodies. If you are with a friend who discusses their appearance in a disparaging way, change the subject or try to shift the focus on to why they are feeling that way, as well as what they can do to improve their body image. Or politely exit the conversation if it is too much to handle.

Finally, if you're struggling with your body image, I have shared a number of my favorite body-positivity websites in the Resources section.

Exercise That Works for *You*

Overcoming your insulin resistance—and improving insulin sensitivity—is not only about modifying and optimizing your diet to stimulate the release of a smaller amount of insulin. A key role is also played by exercise, which improves the sensitivity of one's cells to insulin. Regular exercise reduces central body fat, prevents diabetes, and improves your blood sugar profile by increasing the rate at which muscle cells absorb glucose from the bloodstream (Colberg et al., 2010). The more glucose your body burns during a bout of activity, the longer the body's insulin sensitivity is improved. One study demonstrated that insulin sensitivity improved by 25 percent by increasing exercise from 0 to 60 minutes per day (Nelson et al., 2013).

With these facts in mind, aim to perform at least 30 minutes of exercise every day. To maximize the benefits of exercise, do a combination of aerobic activities and muscle-strengthening exercises.

Sustained aerobic exercise burns calories and glucose during each session and increases the uptake of glucose into cells. Strength training using free weights, machines, and your own body weight will also increase your insulin sensitivity (Van Der Heijden et al., 2010). In addition, strength training helps maintain and build lean muscle mass. Remember, bodies with more muscle mass and less fat tissue generally have higher BMRs. Choose exercises that work all the muscle groups of your body, both in combination and in isolation. Select a weight that challenges you but also allows you to perform three to four sets of 8 to 12 repetitions.

Even if exercise does not immediately show the external changes you desire, don't think your body is not changing internally. One study (Nassis et al., 2005) proved that an insulin sensitivity improvement is possible even without the loss of body weight or fat. Another study (Helmrich, Ragland, Leung, and Paffenbarger, 1991) found that each 500-calorie-per-week increase in energy expenditure reduced one's lifetime risk of type 2 diabetes by 6 percent.

FAQS FOR BUSY PEOPLE WITH LIMITED RESOURCES

Despite an awareness of the numerous benefits of exercise and its crucial role in managing insulin resistance, you may still find it difficult to stick to a regular plan. You are not alone. The following 10 common questions address obstacles you may face when beginning your exercise journey, so take a look at my advice on overcoming these, and get your body moving!

1. What if I'm too busy to exercise?

Work and family commitments may be priorities in your life and likely take up most of your day. The key is to also make exercise a priority. Plan exercise sessions the same way you would schedule an appointment. At the start of the week, map out times you will be able to exercise, and mark them in your diary. It might take a while to find what works for you; it could be a walk at lunch, 10 minutes of strength training before and after work, a weekend hike with your family, or an hour in the evening at the gym. Do not let anything that isn't a matter of urgency derail you from your exercise plans.

2. What if I hate exercising?

Exercise does not have to be a miserable experience. If you hate running, there is no reason to force yourself to do it every day. Walking with a friend in the park or around the neighborhood to see the changes of the seasons may be more your style. You will find it much easier to stick to your plan if you partake in enjoyable forms of exercise. You might discover you enjoy aerobic dancing, swimming, rock climbing, tennis—even pole dancing. Be sure to begin your new exercise routine at a level your body can handle, so you'll want to do it again.

3. What should I do if I lack motivation?

Sometimes you may have the time and resources to exercise, but lack the motivation to follow through. You might get home from work with the best intentions, but find yourself putting on your pajamas instead of hitting the gym. How to avoid avoiding exercise? First, pack a bag with a change of clothes, so after work you can go straight to the gym or wherever you choose to exercise. Second, find someone to keep you accountable. If you have a friend who is waiting to walk with you or a buddy who is saving you a bike in spin class, you'll be less likely to blow off exercising for a night napping on the couch. Third, try practicing self-compassion. Research has shown that practicing self-compassion cultivates the motivation we need to engage in healthy behaviors.

4. How can I exercise when I'm too tired?

I get it: At the end of a long day, the last thing you want to do is lace up your running shoes. Surprisingly, one of the most effective things you can do to increase your energy level is to exercise more. Focus on how much better you will feel afterward. When possible, schedule activities for the times you feel most energetic: Try waking up earlier to work out first thing in the morning, or exercise on your lunch break.

5. What if I can't afford a gym membership?

You do not need a gym membership to exercise. You can walk, run, or cycle outside, and you can perform workouts in the comfort of your own home using nothing more than your own body weight. The basic exercise plans on pages 44 and 45 do not require any equipment at all. Or, if you prefer, you can invest in a jump rope and some basic strength equipment, such as resistance bands and a couple of sets of dumbbells.

6. Do I need a personal trainer?

Having a personal trainer will certainly help if you are new to the gym and want to learn how to perform certain exercises—particularly those involving free weights—correctly. But a trainer isn't essential. Many people teach themselves proper exercise form by reading magazines and watching instructional YouTube videos.

7. How do I exercise when I hate the way my body looks?

When you are getting started, you may feel uncomfortable. If you are overweight, you may feel out of place in a gym and think everyone is mocking you. The truth is, nobody pays attention to anyone but themselves when they are working out. In addition, everyone has to start somewhere; that super fit guy pumping out bicep curls wasn't born that way. You will gain the respect of fellow gym members simply by showing up. But if you feel too uncomfortable, try visiting the gym at nonpeak hours or starting with home workouts.

8. What if my family/friends are not supportive?

Tell your friends and family how important it is to your health to exercise regularly, and ask for their support and encouragement. Better yet, invite them to join you in your activities. You might start a new family tradition of walking together on Saturday mornings. You can also strike up new friendships with physically active people by joining a walking group or dance class.

9. What should I do if my previous attempts at exercise have always failed?

Many people go from 0 to 100 overnight when they start an exercise routine, and wonder why they fail. If you haven't exercised in a while, do not suddenly commit to daily two-hour workouts. Start small and set realistic goals, such as walking for 15 to 20 minutes most days per week. Once you succeed in hitting your small goals consistently, make them a little more challenging.

10. How can I minimize my risk of injury?

Learn how to warm up and cool down to prevent injury, and select exercises appropriate for your fitness level, age, and health status. Taking group fitness classes is an economical way to learn proper exercise technique. Again, take care not to ramp up your exercise intensity and frequency too quickly. Start with low-risk activities such as walking and swimming. If you have any existing health conditions, make sure you are cleared by your physician before embarking on a new exercise regime.

INTUITIVE EATING

Once you have made it through the 28-day meal plan, your body will be free of refined sugars, white flours, and the most dangerous fats. By this time you should be (hopefully) well into your new exercise regime, and feeling healthier and more energetic than ever.

As you move away from the meal plan, you can start trying to eat intuitively. What this means is eating according to your natural hunger and satiety signals, rather than following a plan or consuming a particular number of calories.

BASIC EXERCISE PLANS

The following are four exercise plans and a body-weight resistance training workout that you can do anytime, anywhere—no gym membership required.

› **15-minute option:** If you only have 15 minutes, the best exercise is a brisk walk to get the blood flowing throughout your whole body.

› **30-minute option:** With slightly more available time, walk for 15 minutes, then perform 15 minutes of a circuit of body-weight resistance exercises (see descriptions below). Perform as many push-ups as possible, followed by 12 air squats, 12 tricep dips, and 20 walking lunges. Repeat the whole circuit two more times, for three sets total, resting for 90 to 120 seconds between them. Keep rest to a minimum between individual exercises.

› **45-minute option:** Again, walk for 15 minutes, then devote 30 minutes to the first 10 exercises of the body-weight resistance training workout below. Instead of performing the resistance exercises as a circuit, this time do straight sets. This means perform all the sets of one exercise, then rest for 45 to 60 seconds before moving on to the next series.

› **60-minute option:** With a full hour available, walk for 20 minutes at a brisk pace. Then complete the entire body-weight resistance training workout laid out below.

BODY-WEIGHT RESISTANCE TRAINING WORKOUT

› **Air Squats—3 x 12 repetitions:** Stand with your feet hip-width apart and your arms extended straight in front of you. Push your hips back, squat until your thighs are just past parallel to the ground, and then return to standing.

› **Jumping Jacks—3 x 30 seconds:** Stand with your feet together and hands by your sides. Jump your feet apart, while clapping your hands over your head. Jump again to return to the original position, and repeat as many times as possible within the time limit.

› **Push-ups—3 x as many repetitions as possible:** Place your hands on the floor, shoulder-width apart, and extend your legs behind you. Lower your chest to about 1 inch above the ground, and push yourself back up, while squeezing your stomach muscles to keep your body in a straight line.

› **Burpees—3 x 10 repetitions:** Stand with your feet shoulder-width apart. Push your hips back and squat all the way to the floor, placing your hands on the ground and jumping your feet back to assume a push-up position. Reverse the motion to return to standing. (This is one repetition.)

› **Tricep Dips—3 x as many repetitions as possible:** Place your hands on a bench, chair, or step behind you, and walk your feet forward. Keep your knees bent, then try straightening your legs to increase the difficulty. Lower your body until your upper arms are parallel to the ground, then use your triceps to push yourself back up.

› **High Knees—3 x 30 seconds:** Run on the spot, raising your knees above hip level while pumping your arms.

› **Single-Leg Glute Bridge—3 x 10 repetitions per side:** Lie on your back on the floor, with your knees bent. Lift one leg straight up in the air, then raise your hips until your body is in a straight line, squeeze your glutes, and slowly lower your hips.

› **Plank—3 x 30 seconds:** Get into a similar position to a push-up, but rest your elbows on the floor. Brace your core muscles, and hold your body in a straight line.

› **Walking Lunges—3 x 20 steps:** Step forward with one leg tracking in front of the other, and lower yourself until your back knee is about 1 inch from the ground and your front thigh is parallel to the floor. As you return to standing, step forward with the other leg, and lower yourself toward the ground.

› **Mountain Climbers—3 x 30 seconds:** Begin in a push-up position. Bring one knee toward your chest, then explosively change legs. Keep alternating as quickly as possible.

› **Split Squats—3 x 8 repetitions per side:** Extend one foot behind your body—almost resembling a lunge position, but elevating your back foot on a step or bench. Lower yourself until your rear knee almost touches the ground, and then return to standing. Keep your torso upright and keep your front knee in line with your front foot throughout the movement.

› **Wall Sit—3 x 30 seconds:** Imagine you're sitting in a straight-backed chair. Start with your back against a wall, and set your feet shoulder-width apart about two feet from the wall. Carefully slide your back down the wall until your thighs are parallel to the ground, and try to maintain a squat position. Ensure that your back is flat against the wall and that your hips and knees form a right angle. Your knees should be in line with your ankles and not bent over your toes. The goal is to hold this position for 30 seconds, or as long as you're able to.

When your body feels hungry, feed it nutritious foods. Once you have eliminated unhealthy foods from your system, your body should—in theory—be able to maintain a healthy weight naturally while you eat intuitively.

Because hunger levels are higher when you are insulin resistant, they may not be reliable signals of actual hunger during the early days of following the Insulin Resistance Diet. It takes time for your brain to receive the message that insulin has been released and food is digesting. You cannot expect years of dysfunctional eating habits and the associated imbalances in brain chemistry to be immediately reversed after following a 28-day meal plan. Be patient, and stick with the plan as long as necessary before attempting to eat intuitively.

Intuitive eating is not only about tuning in to hunger and satiety levels but also about tuning in to your moods, especially as emotion can mimic feelings of hunger. Practicing mindfulness will help you understand true hunger. Many people eat simply because they think they are hungry, when in fact they are actually thirsty or even just bored.

I learned to overcome my own emotional eating by finding other non-food-related activities to engage in: I would try calling a friend or going for a walk when I suspected I might be mistaking boredom for hunger, or I would stretch while watching television to prevent mindless snacking. My suggestion is to drink a large glass of water whenever you think you are hungry, and then wait 15 to 20 minutes. At this point, if you still feel hungry, it is true hunger, and time for you to eat.

Make sure you have healthy food on hand. You want to fuel your body appropriately, rather than "intuitively" eating a whole pint of ice cream. An important part of intuitive eating is evaluating how you feel after consuming a certain food. You are likely to feel a whole lot better in terms of energy, mood, and digestion after you've eaten proteins and vegetables, like steak and salad, than high-glycemic carbs, like pizza and donuts.

When you feel ready to eat intuitively, I suggest starting with a 14-day trial, during which you eat according to your hunger levels. During this trial stage, write down everything you consume. Weigh yourself before and after the period. Based on whether you lose, gain, or maintain weight, use your food diary to revise your caloric intake upward or downward as necessary. Then, try eating intuitively without tracking your food in any way.

TROUBLESHOOTING GUIDE

The following common problems may feel like stumbling blocks, but don't let them get in your way. There are solutions to keep you moving forward on your journey of intuitive eating and living.

DEALING WITH CRAVINGS: As explained in chapter 1, the longer you go without consuming highly processed foods, the less you will crave them, so stock your fridge and pantry with nutritious foods, and keep healthy snacks on hand. For a long time I struggled with strong cravings for sweets like chocolates, cakes, and ice creams, but I found having one or two squares of dark chocolate per day kept my cravings away. After a month, I no longer craved regular milk chocolate or other desserts.

EATING OUT: Don't feel intimidated by eating out—most restaurants will be able to accommodate your dietary requests. Even if there is nothing on the menu that appears to cater to your needs, most establishments will be happy to grill meat or fish with basic seasoning, and accompany it with fresh vegetables.

EATING DUE TO BOREDOM OR EMOTION: You are not alone if you find yourself turning to food during times of emotional turmoil or mindlessly snacking out of habit. Replace your unhealthy snacks with fruits and vegetables. Distract yourself with non-food-related activities such as walking, yoga, meditation, massage, reading, or a hot bath. These activities include the added benefit of stress relief, which will also help improve your insulin sensitivity.

PEER PRESSURE: Friends and family may try to convince you to indulge in not-so-healthy foods with them, making comments such as "One piece of cake won't hurt you." This is where your intuition comes in. Listen to whether or not you truly want to indulge in that moment, and don't be afraid to politely decline.

INEXPERIENCE WITH COOKING: Many people reach for processed, packaged foods for their convenience. But the fact is that eating to improve your insulin sensitivity can be simple and time-efficient. All the recipes in this book have been designed to be easy to prepare!

EXPENSE OF COOKING: Many people assume that eating healthy is expensive. However, even when increasing their meat and vegetable spending, with the elimination of spending money on processed foods, the grocery bill should balance out. There are many ways to eat healthy on a budget, too, such as buying in bulk, planning meals in advance, choosing in-season produce, and freezing both perishable bulk foods and leftovers.

DISLIKE OF VEGETABLES: When your taste buds are accustomed to overly salty and sweet processed foods, they may not initially enjoy vegetables. Begin your journey into the joys of eating veggies by not overcooking or under-seasoning them. There are many flavorful ways to prepare vegetables, as you will find in the recipes to follow.

IDEAL BEVERAGES: Although plain water is the recommended choice of beverage for those with insulin resistance, water can get boring. Some alternative low- to zero-calorie options include green tea, herbal tea (my favorites are peppermint and chamomile), and coconut water. You might also try making your own infused water with cucumber, ginger, lemon, lime, mint, or orange. My personal favorite is combining cucumber, mint, and orange for a zingy and refreshing burst of flavor.

UNREALISTIC GOALS: Remember, you cannot expect to follow a diet perfectly the rest of your life. Off-plan meals do not have to be "slip-ups," but can be a part of your life in moderation. Setting unrealistic goals will only make you more likely to abandon the plan the moment you face an obstacle.

WEIGHT-LOSS PLATEAUS: If you are trying to lose weight while eating intuitively, you will almost inevitably reach a point where your weight loss will stall. When you hit that plateau, keep a food diary for seven days. Afterward, decrease your daily caloric intake by 200 to 300 calories to reignite weight loss. I find the most important thing is *not* to give up during this time. Again, remind yourself of all the positive progress you have made already, and focus on forward movement.

MINDFUL EATING AND EATING MEDITATION

Mindful eating is the practice of deliberately paying attention to your thoughts, feelings, and physical sensations while you eat. An acquired skill, it cultivates awareness of what you're doing without feelings of judgment or criticism.

Many people eat in a manner that seems mindless or without conscious thought, or they eat for comfort without really noticing or appreciating their food. This makes it very easy to unconsciously consume hundreds or even thousands of calories' worth of unhealthy food.

Research has shown that eating mindfully can help manage cravings, promote positive eating habits, and encourage the maintenance of a healthy body weight. In a 2006 article for the *Journal of Counseling Psychology*, Tracy Tylka, PhD, noted that people who eat mindfully are more likely to have lower body weights, a greater sense of well-being, and fewer symptoms of eating disorders.

Mindful eating helps you tune into your true feelings of hunger and satiety and increases your understanding of how certain foods affect you. It can also help you address any emotional issues you may have surrounding food and encourage you to choose healthier options.

So, ready to practice a simple eating meditation? Follow the easy steps below.

1. **Enjoy your meal free of distractions, turning off electronic devices.** Plan to just eat.

2. **Give your full attention to the meal in front of you.** Observe the colors and shapes of the food on your plate.

3. **Give thanks.** Acknowledge where the food has come from and express gratitude to those who have prepared each element of the meal.

4. **Take in the aroma of the food, breathing in deeply.**

5. **Select a small piece of food and place it in your mouth.** Let it sit on your tongue as you notice its flavors and textures. Chew carefully, paying attention to how the textures and flavors change.

6. **Swallow and feel the food moving down your throat.** Imagine it traveling throughout your body, nourishing and healing your cells.

7. **Continue taking small bites and chewing slowly, setting down your utensil between each bite.** This will not only improve your digestion and increase your awareness of hunger and satiety, but it will also help you savor each bite.

8. **Listen to your body's signals and stop eating when you feel full, even if your plate is not empty.**

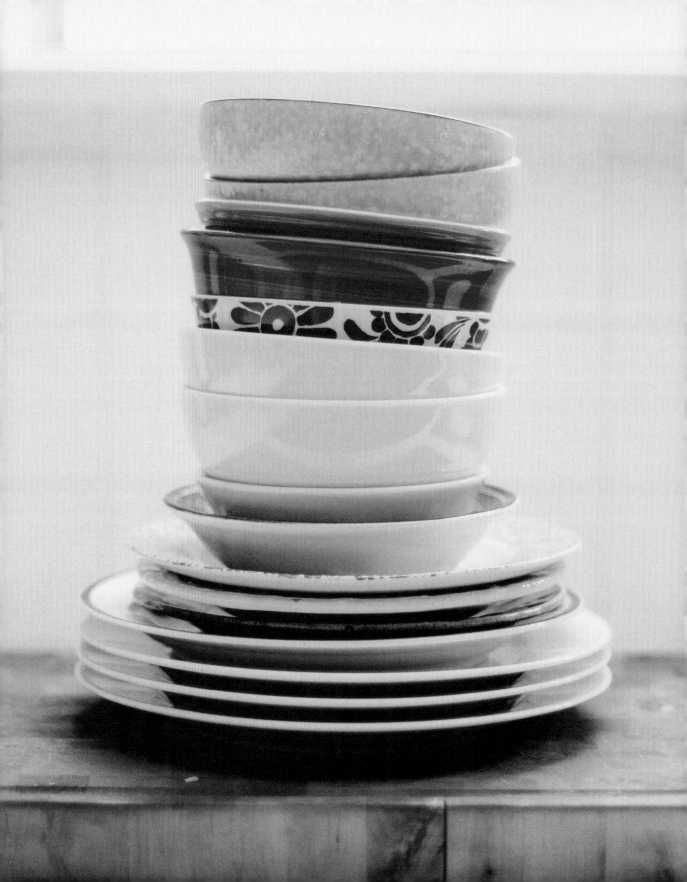

CHAPTER THREE

The Insulin Resistance Diet Meal Plan

Once you've been inspired to make dietary changes to improve your health, where and how should you begin? This chapter outlines every meal you will eat for the next 28 days, including the equipment you may need and pantry staples you should stock up on to start making the simple and delicious recipes featured in the meal plan. The clear instructions offered here will make it easy for you to take charge of your health and overcome your insulin resistance.

One Month to a Healthier Diet

People who are fit and healthy don't usually get that way because of genetics or good luck. Much more likely is that they have formed successful habits. Following the 28-day meal plan is the beginning of new dietary practices that you can sustain for life. Remember to be patient; it is unrealistic to expect to reverse a medical condition in only one month. It may take several months to reestablish normal levels of insulin sensitivity.

Even so, you should see an improvement in your overall symptoms almost immediately. Focus on the positive changes in your energy levels, moods, digestion, weight loss, and relationship with your body image. Paying attention to what's working makes it easy to stick with your new habits long after the 28-day plan is over.

Each time you stick to your plan instead of giving in to temptation, you strengthen your willpower. You also further ingrain your new lifestyle. Sooner than you think, you will find yourself automatically reaching for healthier food options, rather than wrestling with taste buds that beg you to eat junk food. Where you once grasped at excuses to avoid going to the gym, you'll discover exercise becoming a natural part of your everyday life. With time, your new healthy eating and general living habits will enable you to conquer your insulin resistance.

The meal plan and recipes on the following pages eliminate the foods that have been making your insulin resistance worse. The plan and recipes are designed to make forming new routines as simple and convenient as possible. No meal will take longer than 15 minutes to prepare, and all of the ingredients are not only healthy but also affordable. Time spent in the kitchen is minimized: Many of the recipes provide leftovers for subsequent meals, and many weekend meals are prepared in bulk quantities. Finally, all the recipes in this book produce tasty dishes. You may even discover new favorite foods that increase your intake of the nutrients you need and help you maintain healthy practices for life.

SHOPPING GUIDE

Shopping for food when following a nutrition plan can be challenging, especially when you first change your diet. Sourcing out the best and most cost-efficient ingredients takes time and genuine commitment. Cooking from scratch with fresh ingredients also means your shopping cart might be fuller, so set up a practical budget to ensure that you stick to your plan. One issue you will likely encounter is that fresh, unprocessed food, especially organic meats and produce, can be expensive, so here are 5 tips for maintaining reasonable costs:

> **Eat locally and seasonally:** This will be easy if you live in an area with abundant crops and livestock. The less distance ingredients need to travel, the lower the cost. Seasonal food is also tastier, more nutritious, and fresher.

> **Shop at farmers' markets or join a community-supported agriculture program (CSA):** Most areas have markets in the spring and summer featuring fruits, vegetables, and meats—a cost-effective source of locally grown ingredients. CSAs are gaining popularity too—after an initial investment you receive a constant stream of freshly grown produce at minimal cost. The only downside is that they send whatever is ripe and ready—not necessarily all the ingredients you need.

> **Bring a list to the grocery store and stick to it:** Missing ingredients for a recipe just means more trips to the store, while grabbing unnecessary items can quickly inflate your bill.

> **Serve vegetarian meals more often:** The biggest expenses on any grocery bill are the meats, poultry, and fish. Vegetarian meals are a fabulous way to trim these costs while still serving delicious meals.

> **Buy in bulk:** Dry goods such as nuts, whole grains, beans, canned goods, spices, and rice noodles are cheaper in larger quantities, so stock up, especially when they are on sale. Don't buy so much, however, that you risk items spoiling, especially spices; check the labels to ensure that the "best before" date is at least 6 months away.

The 4-Week Meal Plan

WEEK 1 MEAL PLAN

	BREAKFAST	LUNCH	DINNER
M	Nutty Steel-Cut Oatmeal with Blueberries (PAGE 84)	Summer Fruit and Greens Salad (PAGE 99)	Marinara-Braised Meatballs (double recipe) (PAGE 176)
T	Green Pear Protein Smoothie (PAGE 187)	Marinara-Braised Meatballs (leftovers)	Red Lentil Curry (double recipe) (PAGE 132)
W	Spinach and Eggs Skillet (PAGE 95)	Red Lentil Curry (leftovers)	Green Curry Mussels (PAGE 144)
T	Pear-Quinoa Hot Cereal (PAGE 85)	Mixed Greens and Egg Salad with Balsamic Vinaigrette (PAGE 105)	Turkey and Bean Chili (double recipe) (PAGE 168)
F	Fennel-Chard Smoothie (PAGE 188)	Turkey and Bean Chili (leftovers)	Zucchini Pasta with Savory Cherry Tomato Sauce (PAGE 138)
S	Asparagus-Scallion Frittata (PAGE 94)	Mediterranean Quinoa Salad (PAGE 98)	Ginger Rice Noodles with Chicken (double recipe) (PAGE 162)
S	Toasty Oatmeal Pancakes (PAGE 87)	Ginger Rice Noodles with Chicken (leftovers)	Greek-Style Lamb Roast (PAGE 174)

Suggested Snacks

Apple Leather (PAGE 120)

Cantaloupe wedges

Garlicky Hummus (PAGE 117)

Pumpkin seeds

Watermelon wedges

WEEK 1 SHOPPING LIST

Fruits and Vegetables

Asparagus (½ pound)
Baby greens (6 cups)
Blueberries (1 cup)
Cantaloupe (1)
Carrots (4)
Cherry tomatoes (6 cups)
English cucumber (1)
Fennel (1 bulb)
Garlic (1 head)
Ginger (6-inch piece)
Jalapeño peppers (2)
Leek (1)
Lemons (3)
Limes (4)
Onions (6)
Orange (1)
Peach (1)
Pears (3)
Radishes (5)
Red apples (5)
Red bell peppers (2)
Red onion (1)
Scallions (8)
Snow peas (4 cups)
Spinach (24 ounces)
Tomatoes (30 or 5 [28-ounce] cans sodium-free diced tomatoes)
Watercress (5 cups)
Watermelon (1)
Yellow bell pepper (1)
Zucchini (4)

Dairy, Dairy Alternatives, and Eggs

Almond milk, unsweetened (1 half-gallon)
Coconut milk, unsweetened (1 half-gallon)
Coconut milk, light (1 [14-ounce] can)
Eggs (18)

Fresh Herbs

Basil (1 bunch)
Cilantro (1 bunch)
Oregano (1 bunch)
Parsley (1 bunch)
Tarragon (1 bunch)
Thyme (1 bunch)

Seafood

Mussels (1 pound)

Meat and Poultry

Beef, lean ground (1 pound)
Chicken breasts, boneless, skinless (4 [5-ounce] breast halves)
Lamb leg (2 pounds)
Pork, lean ground (1 pound)
Turkey breast, lean ground (2 pounds)

Pantry Items

Almond butter
Almond flour
Almonds, slivered (1 cup)
Almonds, whole (½ cup)
Apple cider vinegar
Baking powder
Baking soda
Balsamic vinegar
Bay leaf
Black beans (2 [14-ounce] cans)
Cayenne
Chicken broth, low sodium (3 cups)
Chickpeas (2 [14-ounce] cans)
Chili powder
Clam juice (1 4-ounce] bottle)
Coconut oil
Dijon mustard
Freshly ground black pepper
Green curry paste
Ground cinnamon
Ground cloves
Ground cumin
Ground ginger
Ground nutmeg
Oats, rolled
Olive oil
Peanuts (6 tablespoons)
Pumpkin seeds (2 tablespoons)
Quinoa (2 cups)
Red curry paste
Red kidney beans (2 [14-ounce] cans)
Red lentils (3 cups)
Red pepper flakes
Rice noodles, dried (8 ounces)
Sea salt
Steel-cut oats (1 cup)
Sun-dried tomatoes (½ cup)
Turmeric
Vanilla extract, pure
Vegetable broth, low sodium (11 cups)
White balsamic vinegar

WEEK 2 MEAL PLAN

	BREAKFAST	LUNCH	DINNER
M	Spinach and Eggs Skillet **(PAGE 95)**	Greek-Style Lamb Roast (leftovers)	Stuffed Tomatoes **(PAGE 136)**
T	Summer Vegetable Smoothie **(PAGE 189)**	Quinoa Lemon Salad **(PAGE 102)**	Chicken Vegetable Meatloaf (double recipe) **(PAGE 163)**
W	Nutty Steel-Cut Oatmeal with Blueberries **(PAGE 84)**	Chicken Vegetable Meatloaf (leftovers)	Pistachio-Crusted Salmon **(PAGE 154)**
T	Creamy Green Apple Smoothie **(PAGE 190)**	Mediterranean Quinoa Salad **(PAGE 98)**	Red Lentil Curry (double recipe) **(PAGE 132)**
F	Asparagus-Scallion Frittata **(PAGE 94)**	Red Lentil Curry (leftovers)	Braised Pork Cutlets with Spinach (double recipe) **(PAGE 169)**
S	Toasty Oatmeal Pancakes **(PAGE 87)**	Braised Pork Cutlets with Spinach (leftovers)	Shrimp and Mussel Paella (double recipe) **(PAGE 147)**
S	Vegetable Baked Eggs **(PAGE 92)**	Shrimp and Mussel Paella (leftovers)	Roast Beef with Wild Mushroom Sauce **(PAGE 180)**

Suggested Snacks

Almonds

Apple Leather **(PAGE 120)**

Guacamole Dip **(PAGE 116)**

Hardboiled egg

Vegetable crudités

WEEK 2 SHOPPING LIST

Fruits and Vegetables

Avocado (1)

Blueberries (1 cup)

Butternut squash (1)

Chanterelle mushrooms
    (4 ounces)

Cherry tomatoes (1 cup)

English cucumber (1)

Garlic (1 head)

Ginger (6-inch piece)

Green apples (2)

Kale (1 bunch)

Leek (1)

Lemons (4)

Onions (4)

Oyster mushrooms (8 ounces)

Red bell peppers (5)

Scallions (4)

Shallots (2)

Shiitake mushrooms (4 ounces)

Snap peas (½ cup)

Spinach (50 ounces)

Tomatoes (14)

Yellow bell pepper (1)

Dairy, Dairy Alternatives, and Eggs

Coconut milk
    (1 [14-ounce] can)

Eggs (7)

Fresh Herbs

Basil (1 bunch)

Cilantro (1 bunch)

Oregano (1 bunch)

Parsley (1 bunch)

Thyme (1 bunch)

Seafood

Mussels (1 pound)

Salmon fillets
    (4 [6-ounce] fillets)

Shrimp, peeled, deveined
    (1 pound, 16 to 20 count)

Meat and Poultry

Chicken, lean ground
    (2 pounds)

Pork chops, boneless
    (8 [4-ounce] chops)

Sirloin tip beef roast (1 pound)

Pantry Items

Almond butter

Almonds, ground

Almonds, slivered (½ cup)

Almonds, whole (½ cup)

Apple cider vinegar

Brown rice (1 cup)

Cayenne

Chicken broth, low sodium
    (4 cups)

Dijon mustard

Freshly ground black pepper

Green lentils
    (1 [14-ounce] can)

Ground cinnamon

Ground cumin

Ground ginger

Ground nutmeg

Olive oil

Pistachios, dry-roasted,
    unsalted (1 cup)

Quinoa (2 cups)

Red curry paste

Red lentils (3 cups)

Saffron threads

Sea salt

Steel-cut oats (1 cup)

Sunflower seeds (½ cup)

Turmeric

Vegetable broth, low sodium
    (10 cups)

3

WEEK 3 MEAL PLAN

	BREAKFAST	LUNCH	DINNER
M	Pear-Quinoa Hot Cereal **(PAGE 85)**	Mixed Greens and Egg Salad with Balsamic Vinaigrette **(PAGE 105)**	Vegetable Stew (double recipe) **(PAGE 135)**
T	Asparagus-Scallion Frittata **(PAGE 94)**	Vegetable Stew (leftovers)	Tender Crab Cakes **(PAGE 145)**
W	Green Pear Protein Smoothie **(PAGE 187)**	Wheat Berry–Grape Salad (double recipe) **(PAGE 100)**	Breaded Chicken with Mustard **(PAGE 165)**
T	Fennel-Chard Smoothie **(PAGE 188)**	Wheat Berry–Grape Salad (leftovers)	Marinara-Braised Meatballs (double recipe) **(PAGE 176)**
F	Nutty Steel-Cut Oatmeal with Blueberries **(PAGE 84)**	Marinara-Braised Meatballs (leftovers)	Veggie Pecan Burgers **(PAGE 133)**
S	Vegetable Baked Eggs **(PAGE 92)**	Chicken Barley Soup **(PAGE 113)**	Shrimp and Mussel Paella (double recipe) **(PAGE 147)**
S	Quinoa Waffles **(PAGE 88)**	Shrimp and Mussel Paella (leftovers)	Greek-Style Lamb Roast (double recipe) **(PAGE 174)**

Suggested Snacks

Apple

Celery with almond butter

Cucumber slices

Garlicky Hummus **(PAGE 117)**

Pesto Veggie Pizza **(PAGE 118)**

WEEK 3 SHOPPING LIST

Fruits and Vegetables

Asparagus (½ pound)
Baby greens (6 cups)
Blueberries (1 cup)
Carrots (6)
Celery stalks (13)
Cherry tomatoes (2 cups)
Eggplant (1)
English cucumber (1)
Fennel (1 head)
Garlic (1 head)
Ginger (3-inch piece)
Green cabbage (1 head)
Green grapes (4 cups)
Kale (2 cups)
Lemons (3)
Limes (2)
Onions (8)
Orange (1)
Peach (1)
Pears (3)
Red apples (2)
Red bell peppers (5)
Red onion (1)
Scallions (6)
Tomatoes (17)
Yellow bell pepper (1)
Zucchini (1)

Dairy, Dairy Alternatives, and Eggs

Almond milk, unsweetened
    (1 half-gallon)
Coconut milk, unsweetened
    (1 half-gallon)

Eggs (20)
Yogurt, plain (¼ cup)

Fresh Herbs

Basil (1 bunch)
Cilantro (1 bunch)
Dill (1 bunch)
Mint (2 bunches)
Oregano (1 bunch)
Parsley (1 bunch)
Tarragon (1 bunch)
Thyme (1 bunch)

Seafood

Lump crabmeat (1 pound)
Mussels (1 pound)
Shrimp, peeled, deveined
    (1 pound, 16 to 20 count)

Meat and Poultry

Beef, lean ground (1 pound)
Chicken breasts, boneless,
    skinless (4 [4-ounce]
    breast halves)
Chicken meat, cooked (3 cups)
Lamb leg (2 pounds)
Pork, lean ground (1 pound)

Pantry Items

Almond butter (3 tablespoons)
Almond flour
Almonds, slivered (1 pound)
Almonds, whole (1 pound)
Apple cider vinegar
Applesauce, unsweetened
Baking powder

Balsamic vinegar
Bay leaf
Brown rice (1 cup)
Chicken broth, low sodium
    (11 cups)
Chickpeas (1 [14-ounce] can)
Coconut oil
Flaxseed (1 teaspoon)
Freshly ground black pepper
Grainy mustard
Ground cinnamon
Ground coriander
Ground cumin
Ground ginger
Ground nutmeg
Honey
Olive oil
Pearl barley (½ cup)
Pecans, chopped (1 cup)
Quinoa (1 cup)
Quinoa flour (1 cup)
Red pepper flakes
Saffron threads
Sea salt
Steel-cut oats
Sunflower seeds (1¼ cups)
Tamari sauce, low sodium
Vanilla extract, pure
Vegetable broth, sodium-free
    (4 cups)
Wheat berries (2 cups)
White balsamic vinegar

WEEK 4 MEAL PLAN

	BREAKFAST	LUNCH	DINNER
M	Creamy Green Apple Smoothie (PAGE 190)	Greek-Style Lamb Roast (leftovers)	Stuffed Tomatoes (PAGE 136)
T	Nutty Steel-Cut Oatmeal with Blueberries (PAGE 84)	Arugula Chicken Salad with Tahini Dressing (PAGE 106)	Nut-Breaded Lemon Cod (PAGE 150)
W	Asparagus-Scallion Frittata (PAGE 94)	Fruited Bean Salad (PAGE 104)	Marinara-Braised Meatballs (double recipe) (PAGE 176)
T	Summer Vegetable Smoothie (PAGE 189)	Marinara-Braised Meatballs (leftovers)	Vegetable Stew (double recipe) (PAGE 135)
F	Pear-Quinoa Hot Cereal (PAGE 85)	Vegetable Stew (leftovers)	Ocean Perch with Citrus-Fennel Slaw (PAGE 153)
S	Quinoa Waffles (PAGE 88)	Green Power Soup (double recipe) (PAGE 111)	Roast Beef with Wild Mushroom Sauce (PAGE 180)
S	Vegetable Baked Eggs (PAGE 92)	Green Power Soup (leftovers)	Artichoke-Chicken Bake (PAGE 164)

Suggested Snacks

Blueberries

Fennel-Chard Smoothie (PAGE 188)

Guacamole Dip (PAGE 116)

Hardboiled egg

Plain yogurt

WEEK 4 SHOPPING LIST

Fruits and Vegetables

Arugula (4 cups)

Asparagus (1 pound)

Avocado (1)

Blueberries (1 cup)

Carrots (4)

Celery stalks (12)

Chanterelle mushrooms
    (4 ounces)

Eggplant (1)

English cucumber (1)

Fennel bulb (1 head)

Garlic (1 head)

Ginger (2-inch piece)

Grapefruit (1)

Green apples (2)

Green beans (2 cups)

Green cabbage (1 head)

Kale (1 bunch)

Leeks (2)

Lemons (3)

Limes (5)

Onions (5)

Orange (1)

Oyster mushrooms (8 ounces)

Peach (1)

Pears (2)

Red bell peppers (5)

Scallions (4)

Shallots (2)

Shiitake mushrooms (4 ounces)

Snap peas (4½ cups)

Spinach (10 ounces)

Tomatoes (20)

Yellow bell pepper (1)

Zucchini (1)

Dairy, Dairy Alternatives, and Eggs

Almond milk, unsweetened
    (1 half-gallon)

Coconut milk, unsweetened
    (1 half-gallon)

Coconut milk (1 [14-ounce] can)

Eggs (18)

Yogurt, plain (1 cup)

Fresh Herbs

Basil (1 bunch)

Cilantro (1 bunch)

Oregano (1 bunch)

Parsley (1 bunch)

Thyme (2 bunches)

Seafood

Cod fillets (4 [6-ounce] fillets)

Ocean perch fillets
    (4 [6-ounce] fillets)

Meat and Poultry

Beef, lean ground (1 pound)

Chicken breasts, boneless,
    skinless (4 [5-ounce]
    breast halves)

Chicken, cooked (3 cups)

Pork, lean ground (1 pound)

Sirloin tip beef roast (1 pound)

Pantry Items

Almond butter

Almond flour

Almonds, slivered (2 cups)

Almonds, whole (½ cup)

Apple cider vinegar

Applesauce, unsweetened

Artichoke hearts
    (1 [8-ounce] jar)

Baking powder, double acting

Balsamic vinegar

Bay leaf

Chicken broth, low sodium
    (13 cups)

Chickpeas (1 [14-ounce] can)

Coconut oil

Freshly ground black pepper

Green lentils (1 [14-ounce] can)

Ground cardamom

Ground cinnamon

Ground coriander

Ground cumin

Ground ginger

Ground nutmeg

Ground turmeric

Honey

Navy beans (1 [14-ounce] can)

Olive oil

Olive oil cooking spray

Pearl barley (1 cup)

Quinoa (1 cup)

Quinoa flour

Red kidney beans
    (1 [14-ounce] can)

Red pepper flakes

Sea salt

Steel-cut oats (1 cup)

Sunflower seeds

Tahini

Vanilla extract, pure

Vegetable broth, sodium-free
    (4 cups)

PANTRY STAPLES

Having a kitchen stocked with foods that suit the Insulin Resistance Diet can be one of the most important strategies for success. When all your choices are healthy ones, it is very difficult to sabotage yourself after a long stressful day. The following list is not comprehensive and you do not have to buy every item, but if something is on sale and nonperishable it makes good sense to stock up when the opportunity arises. Obviously, when stocking your pantry, you should take into account any other dietary conditions or restrictions, such as allergies, blood pressure issues, or whether you have chosen a vegetarian lifestyle.

Make sure the ingredients you buy are the best quality you can afford, and whenever possible, organic or grass-fed. If you are on a tight budget, you might have to make some tough choices about which foods to purchase organic versus which are sufficient when commercially grown or raised. When in doubt, consult the handy list created by the Environmental Working Group, ranking fruits and vegetables by their pesticide loads in a given year (see the Dirty Dozen and Clean Fifteen lists in Appendix C).

Staple Ingredients

Foods to include in your fridge, freezer, and pantry:

› Lots of low-GI vegetables (either fresh or sodium- and additive-free frozen), including artichoke, asparagus, bean sprouts, spinach, kale, Swiss chard, mustard greens, beet greens, dandelion greens, chicory, endive, escarole, mixed baby greens, collard greens, bok choy, broccoli, Brussels sprouts, cabbage, cauliflower, celery, cucumber, fennel, garlic, ginger, kohlrabi, mushrooms, onions, bell peppers, hot peppers, radishes, tomatoes, turnips, and zucchini. Add medium-GI vegetables in moderation, such as beets, carrots, green beans, eggplant, peas, squashes, and sweet potato.

› Lower-GI fruit (either fresh or additive-free frozen), including avocado, strawberries, blueberries, raspberries, cranberries, cherries, peaches, plums, rhubarb, lemon, lime, pears, and apples. Add medium-GI fruit in moderation, such as grapes, kiwifruit, and melon.

› Fresh herbs

› Organic poultry and meats, such as chicken, turkey, beef, lamb, and pork.

> Eggs, preferably naturally fed and/or organic.

> Seafood, such as cod, anchovies, flounder, haddock (Atlantic), perch (ocean), wild salmon, sardines, sole, halibut, clams, mussels, oysters, scallops, shrimp, and calamari.

> Plain unsweetened yogurt and butter in small amounts.

> Pantry items, including canned or dried legumes (black beans, chickpeas, navy beans, lentils, black-eyed peas, kidney beans, and split peas), nut butters, nut flours, walnuts, almonds, flaxseed, pumpkin seeds, chia seeds, sesame seeds, sunflower seeds, dried herbs, spices, olive oil, coconut oil, flaxseed oil, sesame oil, whole grains and pseudo-grains in moderation (brown rice, wheat berries, quinoa, barley, bulgur, spelt, and wild rice), Bragg's liquid aminos, capers, chili paste, dill pickle, hot sauces, mustard, olives, gluten-free low-sodium broths (vegetable, chicken, fish, and vegetable), tomato paste, Sriracha, sun-dried tomatoes, tahini, low-sodium tamari sauce, tomato paste, vinegar (white wine, white balsamic, rice, balsamic, apple cider), rice noodles, sauerkraut, wasabi paste, Worcestershire sauce, unsweetened applesauce, green tea, herbal tea, arrowroot, baking powder, unsweetened cocoa powder, vanilla extract, almond extract, unsweetened almond milk, and coconut milk (canned and from a carton).

Essential Tools and Equipment

Most of the recipes in this book can be prepared with the tools and equipment found in your kitchen right now; however, there are some pieces of equipment that will save you time or are required for a few specific dishes. Some of the equipment and kitchen tools to consider for your kitchen are listed here:

> **Good-quality knives:** Fresh ingredients means you will be doing a lot of chopping and prepping, so invest in a sharp, sturdy knife to make your kitchen time easier. You should probably have a large chef's knife, a medium-size utility knife, and a small paring knife.

> **Nested stainless-steel mixing bowls:** Bowls are crucial for cooking because there are usually prepped ingredients that need mixing, batters to whisk, and salads that need tossing. Get an assortment of sizes so you will have the correct bowl for the task.

> **Measuring cups and spoons:** Cooking can certainly be a dash of this and a pinch of that, but most recipes turn out better if you measure the ingredients accurately. Vegetables, fruit, meats, and fish can be a little less precisely measured, but sauce ingredients and anything to do with baking need to be more exact.

> **Cutting board:** You do not need dedicated cutting boards for produce, poultry, fish, and red meat like most professional restaurants, but at least two good-size boards are optimal. If you do not have dedicated boards, make sure you scrub your used boards very well to avoid cross-contamination.

> **Saucepans and a stockpot:** Sauces, soups, stews, and many other dishes require different saucepans. Using a large saucepan for a sauce that specifies a small saucepan will affect the cooking time and end product, so have large, medium, and small saucepans. This will contribute to culinary success.

> **Nonstick skillets:** You will probably use a large (9- to 10-inch) skillet for many recipes, especially if you are feeding a family of four. A nonstick coating is helpful because you can use less oil, and there is less chance of food sticking and burning.

> **Baking dishes:** Casseroles, baked and braised poultries and meats, and cakes require glass or metal baking dishes. Try to have at least one 9-by-13-inch and one 8-by-8-inch baking dish for various recipes.

> **Baking sheets:** Full-size and half-size baking sheets are crucial for cookies, schnitzels, roasting vegetables and meats, dehydrating, and pizzas. Baking sheets with a 1-inch lip are convenient so that any juices stay on the sheets and do not end up pooled in the bottom of an oven.

> **Food processor:** A food processor is an incredible tool for saving time. This device chops vegetables, purées soups and sauces, mixes dough, and very effectively blends nut butters, flours, and milks.

> **Blender or immersion blender:** A blender a wonderful tool, especially if you don't have a food processor or juicer. An immersion blender is a handheld blending tool that is perfect for smaller quantities of foods. Both are used for puréeing soups, making smoothies, and blending homemade dips and dressings.

> **Grill:** Cooking on a grill is wonderful for meats, poultry, fish, and vegetables, creating a lightly charred result with amazing flavor.

> **Ice cream maker:** You can spend hundreds of dollars on a high-end ice cream maker, or a great deal less on appliances that have simple rotating sections and require rock salt. Ice cream makers create delectable ice cream, sorbets, and sherbets.

> **Waffle iron:** This is an appliance that can create some scrumptious meals very quickly. Homemade waffles are healthier than store-bought versions, and allow you to use ingredients that suit the Insulin Resistance Diet.

Final Encouragement

Supplied with a thorough meal plan, shopping and equipment lists, and quick and easy recipes, you now have all the tools necessary to kickstart your new lifestyle. Remind yourself of the benefits of following the Insulin Resistance Diet not only for your physical health, but also for your emotional well-being and body image. Remember that by eating more natural and healthy foods, you will not only overcome your insulin resistance—and simultaneously manage your PCOS, metabolic syndrome, prediabetes or type 2 diabetes, and weight—but you will feel healthier and more energetic overall. You will become more in tune with your body than ever before. If you are serious about taking charge of your health, the time to act is now.

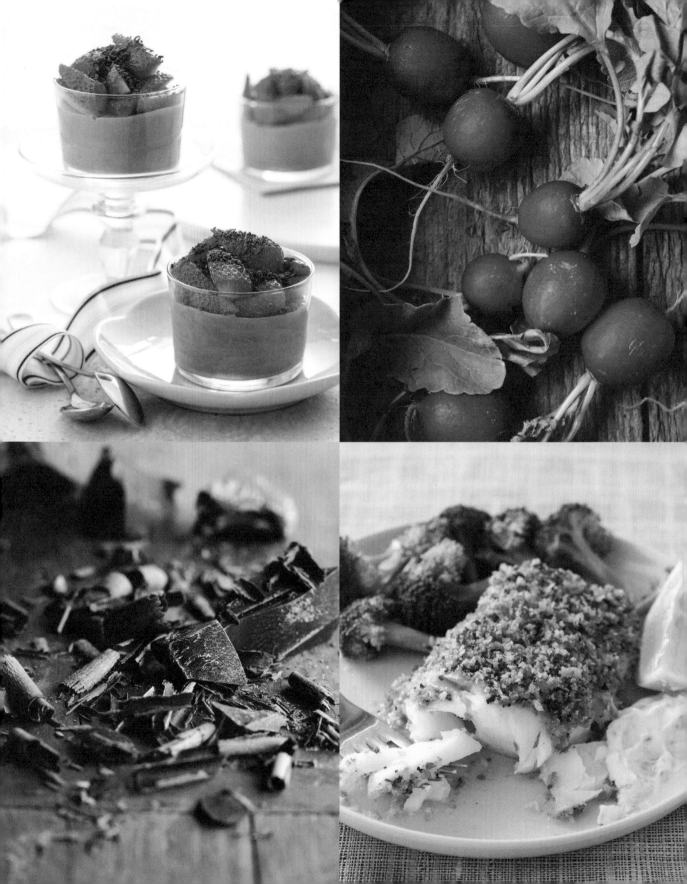

PART II

The
Recipes

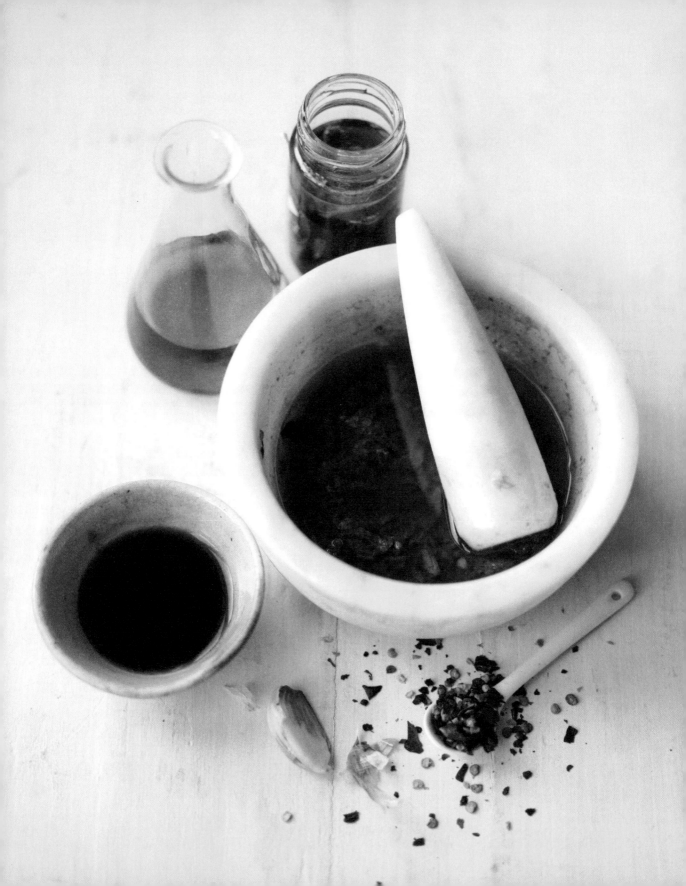

CHAPTER FOUR
Condiments and Stocks

CARIBBEAN JERK RUB

PREP TIME: 5 MINUTES

MAKES ½ CUP

Sometimes deciding what to make for dinner takes longer than actually preparing the meal. When you are exhausted and short on inspiration, sprinkle a little of this spice mix on chicken breasts or pork chops, then grill or bake them, and serve with a fresh tossed salad for a tasty and convenient meal.

2 tablespoons garlic powder

1 tablespoon dried thyme

1 tablespoon onion flakes

2 teaspoons ground allspice

1 teaspoon ground cinnamon

1 teaspoon ground nutmeg

1 teaspoon sea salt

1 teaspoon freshly ground black pepper

1 teaspoon cayenne

1. Stir all the ingredients together in a small bowl until well blended.

2. Store the spice mixture in a sealed jar at room temperature.

> **SERVING TIP:** This seasoning can be used to enhance almost any ingredients, including steak, poultry, seafood, and even vegetables. Jerk rubs contain a fiery kick, so if you prefer a bit less heat, reduce the cayenne to ¼ teaspoon.

PER SERVING (1 teaspoon) Calories: 5; Carbs: 1g; Glycemic Load: 0; Fiber: 0g; Protein: 0g; Sodium: 78mg; Fat: 0g

SESAME VINAIGRETTE

PREP TIME: 10 MINUTES

MAKES 1¼ CUPS

Sesame oil and tahini ensure that this dressing is rich and flavorful, highlighting the toasty luxuriousness of this healthy seed. Try the vinaigrette with shredded kale, snow peas, and sweet chunks of peach for a superb start to a light meal. For an exotic twist, try using this vinaigrette as a marinade for firm white fish.

½ cup rice vinegar

¼ cup freshly squeezed lime juice

¼ cup tahini

2 tablespoons grated fresh ginger

2 tablespoons sesame oil

2 tablespoons low-sodium tamari sauce

2 teaspoons minced garlic

1 teaspoon honey

1. Put all the ingredients in a blender, and purée until smooth.

2. Add a little water if you want a thinner vinaigrette.

3. Store the vinaigrette in a sealed container in the refrigerator for up to 2 weeks.

INGREDIENT TIP: Tahini is a thick paste with an incredibly rich flavor that is enhanced when this ingredient is made with toasted sesame seeds. You might not find the toasted version in a mainstream grocery store, but it's often available in Asian markets and health food stores.

PER SERVING (2 tablespoons) Calories: 196; Carbs: 8g; Glycemic Load: 3; Fiber: 2g; Protein: 4g; Sodium: 369mg; Fat: 15g

FRESH BERRY VINAIGRETTE

PREP TIME: 5 MINUTES

MAKES 2 CUPS

A crisp, colorful salad tossed with a berry-spiked vinaigrette would seem to have all the components of a healthy meal or starter. But this vibrant-hued vinaigrette has the extra benefit of apple cider vinegar. Consuming as little as 2 tablespoons a day of vinegar can reduce blood sugar levels between 25 and 50 percent.

½ cup apple cider vinegar

½ cup fresh raspberries, strawberries, or cranberries

1 tablespoon freshly squeezed lemon juice

½ teaspoon chopped fresh thyme

Pinch sea salt

1 cup olive oil

1. Put the vinegar, berries, lemon juice, thyme, and salt in a blender, and blend until puréed, about 30 seconds.

2. Press the berry mixture through a fine-mesh sieve into a small bowl.

3. Whisk in the olive oil until emulsified.

4. Pour the vinaigrette into a sealable jar, and store in the refrigerator for up to 1 week.

INGREDIENT TIP: Fresh, succulent berries are best for this tangy vinaigrette, but if seasonal fruit is not available, you can substitute frozen berries. Make sure you completely defrost the berries, and drain out the extra liquid before adding them to the other ingredients.

PER SERVING (2 tablespoons) Calories: 112; Carbs: 0g; Glycemic Load: 0; Fiber: 0g; Protein: 0g; Sodium: 16mg; Fat: 13g

CHILE-ANCHOVY DRESSING

PREP TIME: 10 MINUTES
MAKES 2 CUPS

A spicy dressing is a marvelous addition to many different meals; it can deliver just the right kick to an otherwise plain dish. Chile peppers add the heat to this dressing because they contain a compound called capsaicin. Capsaicin is a potent anti-inflammatory, so it fights the inflammation in the body that contributes to insulin resistance.

7 to 10 anchovy fillets

¾ cup olive oil

½ cup apple cider vinegar

2 teaspoons minced garlic

⅛ teaspoon red pepper flakes

Sea salt

Freshly ground black pepper

1. Put the anchovies, olive oil, vinegar, garlic, and red pepper flakes in a blender, and pulse until emulsified.

2. Season with salt and freshly ground black pepper.

3. Transfer the dressing to a container, and store in the refrigerator for up to 1 week.

SERVING TIP: Many people use spicy dressing on almost every dish, so this healthy homemade version will be a welcome addition to your culinary repertoire. Unlike this one, prepared dressings can contain too much sodium, sugar, and additives that you might want to avoid.

PER SERVING (2 tablespoons) Calories: 54; Carbs: 2g; Glycemic: Load 0; Fiber: 1g; Protein: 1g; Sodium: 121mg; Fat: 0g

WASABI MAYONNAISE

PREP TIME: 10 MINUTES
MAKES 1 CUP

With its buttery texture and distinctive taste, avocado is a fruit you either love or hate. Avocado is high in monounsaturated fat, so it can slow digestion when added to a meal. For practical purposes, slathering a tablespoon or two of this pale green condiment on a whole-grain sandwich can help prevent blood sugar spikes, and it tastes fabulous, too.

1 avocado, peeled and pitted

4 teaspoons wasabi paste

2 tablespoons apple cider vinegar

1 tablespoon freshly squeezed lemon juice

Sea salt

Freshly ground black pepper

1. Put the avocado, wasabi paste, vinegar, and lemon juice in a food processor, and process until smooth, scraping down the sides of the bowl at least once.

2. Season with salt and freshly ground black pepper.

3. Store the wasabi mayonnaise in the refrigerator in a sealed container for up to 1 week.

INGREDIENT TIP: Read the label on the wasabi carefully if you are looking for an authentic product. Most of the wasabi sold outside of Japan is actually colored horseradish, which has a harsher, more burning taste than the real deal. True wasabi is more herbal in flavor, with a smooth finish.

PER SERVING (2 tablespoons) Calories: 61; Carbs: 3g; Glycemic Load: 2; Fiber: 1g; Protein: 1g; Sodium: 33mg; Fat: 6g

BASIL SALSA

PREP TIME: 15 MINUTES
MAKES 3 CUPS

Salsa is fun. Combining colorful vegetables, herbs, citrus, and a touch of heat, salsa works equally well as a snack or a simple topping. Chopping the ingredients can be a soothing experience when you need a break from a stressful day. Take the time to inhale the sweet fragrance of the tomatoes before chopping them up.

2 tomatoes, finely chopped

½ yellow bell pepper, finely chopped

½ cup finely chopped English cucumber

½ cup finely chopped sweet onion

½ cup chopped fresh basil

½ jalapeño pepper, finely chopped

2 tablespoons freshly squeezed lime juice

Sea salt

Freshly ground black pepper

1. In a medium bowl, stir together the tomatoes, bell pepper, cucumber, onion, basil, jalapeño pepper, and lime juice until well blended.

2. Season with salt and freshly ground black pepper.

3. Store the salsa in a sealed container in the refrigerator for up to 1 week.

SERVING TIP: Although salsa makes a delicious healthy snack when you have the munchies, it also makes a perfect topper for fish, chicken, and soups. Use an entire jalapeño pepper in the salsa if you like a little more heat.

PER SERVING (¼ cup) Calories: 14; Carbs: 3g; Glycemic Load: 0; Fiber: 1g; Protein: 0g; Sodium: 34mg; Fat: 0g

4

SIMPLE TOMATO SAUCE

PREP TIME: 5 MINUTES • COOK TIME: 45 MINUTES
SERVES 6

If you have only experienced salty jarred tomato sauce, you have missed the absolute joy of creating a bright tomato sauce from scratch. Tomato sauce represents the crowning culinary achievement in many ethnic kitchens—transforming simple ingredients into an extraordinary sauce takes skill. To bring out a more assertive tomato flavor, add a couple of tablespoons of tomato paste along with the herbs.

1 tablespoon olive oil

1 large sweet onion, chopped

4 teaspoons minced garlic

1 carrot, chopped

8 tomatoes, chopped

1 tablespoon apple cider vinegar

1 tablespoon chopped fresh basil

1 tablespoon chopped fresh oregano

1 teaspoon chopped fresh thyme

Pinch red pepper flakes

Sea salt

Freshly ground black pepper

4

1. Put a medium saucepan over medium heat, and add the olive oil.

2. Sauté the onion and garlic until the vegetables are translucent, about 4 minutes.

3. Add the carrot, tomatoes, and vinegar to the saucepan, and bring the mixture to a simmer.

4. Simmer for about 25 minutes, until the carrot chunks are soft.

5. Transfer the tomato mixture to a food processor, and purée until the sauce is smooth.

6. Return the sauce to the saucepan, and stir in the basil, oregano, thyme, and red pepper flakes.

7. Simmer the sauce for 15 minutes to mellow the flavors.

8. Season the sauce with salt and freshly ground black pepper.

9. Serve immediately or cool the sauce completely, and store in a sealed container in the refrigerator for up to 4 days, or in the freezer for up to 1 month.

INGREDIENT TIP: Fresh tomatoes are a healthy choice in recipes, but sometimes canned are the most convenient option when produce is not in season or simply too expensive. If you cannot find seasonal field tomatoes bursting with flavor, look for an organic, sodium-free canned product instead.

PER SERVING (¼ cup) Calories: 70; Carbs: 11g; Glycemic Load: 3; Fiber: 3g; Protein: 2g; Sodium: 56mg; Fat: 3g

HOMEMADE CHICKEN STOCK

PREP TIME: 15 MINUTES · COOK TIME: 22 HOURS
MAKES 8 TO 10 CUPS

Professional kitchens keep a cauldron-size stockpot on a back stove, hidden from view. This pot simmers all day and night, producing gallons of homemade chicken stock for all the soups, sauces, and main courses the kitchen produces. Making your own stock at home is a great way to avoid all the additives, sugar, and sodium found in commercially prepared stocks.

2 chicken carcasses

1 tablespoon apple cider vinegar

3 celery stalks, cut into quarters

2 sweet onions, peeled and quartered

2 carrots, peeled and roughly chopped

4 garlic cloves, smashed

3 fresh thyme sprigs

2 bay leaves

INGREDIENT TIP: Whenever you serve a roasted chicken, save the carcass for this stock after the meat has been stripped off. Carcasses freeze well, so seal them in freezer bags until you have enough to create the stock.

PER SERVING (1 cup) Calories: 78; Carbs: 8g; Glycemic Load: 5; Fiber: 0g; Protein: 6g; Sodium: 245mg; Fat: 1g

1. Preheat the oven to 350°F.

2. Put the carcasses in a baking pan, and roast for 30 minutes, turning once.

3. Transfer the carcasses to a large stockpot, and add the vinegar and enough cold water to cover the carcasses by at least 3 inches.

4. Put the pot over high heat, and bring the stock to a boil.

5. Reduce the heat to low and gently simmer the stock for 12 hours, stirring every few hours.

6. Add the celery, onions, carrots, garlic, thyme, and bay leaves and continue to simmer for 8 hours longer, stirring several times.

7. Remove the pot from the heat, and cool for at least 30 minutes.

8. Remove any large bones with tongs, then strain the stock through a fine-mesh sieve, and discard the solids.

9. Pour the stock into jars that can be sealed, and allow it to cool completely.

10. Seal the jars and store the stock in the refrigerator for up to 5 days, or in the freezer for up to 3 months.

SAVORY BEEF STOCK

PREP TIME: 15 MINUTES • COOK TIME: 21 HOURS

MAKES 8 TO 10 CUPS

The next time you make homemade stock, create batches in handy containers to keep in your freezer. Making stock yourself keeps it free of harmful additives such as gluten, sugar, and sodium. To make glossy, rich demi-glace, put the strained stock back on the stove over low heat, and reduce it by about two-thirds. You can freeze it in ice cube trays for making incredible sauces later on.

3 pounds beef bones

2 tablespoons apple cider vinegar

2 sweet onions, peeled and quartered

2 carrots, peeled and roughly chopped

2 celery stalks, roughly chopped

3 fresh thyme sprigs

½ teaspoon black peppercorns

1. Preheat the oven to 350°F.

2. Put the bones in a baking pan and roast them in the oven for 45 minutes, turning them once with tongs.

3. Transfer the roasted bones to a large stockpot, and add the apple cider vinegar and enough cold water to cover the bones by at least 3 inches.

4. Put the pot over high heat, and bring to a boil.

5. Reduce the heat to low and simmer the beef stock for 12 hours. In the first few hours, check the stock every half hour for impurities floating on the top of the liquid. Skim the impurities off the top with a spoon.

6. Add the onions, carrots, celery, thyme, and peppercorns to the pot, and continue to simmer the stock for 8 hours. ▸▸

7. Remove the pot from the heat and cool slightly.

8. Remove any large bones with tongs, then strain the stock through a fine-mesh sieve, and discard the solids.

9. Pour the stock into jars that have sealable lids, and allow it to cool completely.

10. Seal the jars and store the stock in the refrigerator for up to 5 days, or in the freezer for up to 3 months.

INGREDIENT TIP: If you can't imagine where to find beef bones, don't despair—they are as close as the meat counter at your local grocery store or butcher. With the rise in popularity of bone broth, most stores keep bags of beef bones on hand for their clients, either fresh or frozen.

PER SERVING (1 cup) Calories: 42; Carbs: 3g; Glycemic Load: 3; Fiber: 0g; Protein: 5g; Sodium: 289mg; Fat: 0g

HERBED VEGETABLE STOCK

PREP TIME: 20 MINUTES • COOK TIME: 2 HOURS
MAKES 8 CUPS

A perfect vegetable stock can be sipped as a light snack and should have a delicate herbal taste. You might be surprised at how satisfying it can be when you need an energy boost. The trick is to simmer the vegetables until they are tender but not mushy. If the vegetables break down, you will end up with a murky, unappetizing-looking liquid rather than a clear golden stock.

1 gallon water

5 carrots, cut into large chunks

5 celery stalks, with the greens, cut into chunks

5 garlic cloves, smashed

4 leeks, white and green parts, cut into chunks and cleaned very well

4 tomatoes, quartered

2 sweet onions, peeled and cut into quarters

8 fresh thyme sprigs

8 fresh parsley sprigs

8 whole cloves

2 bay leaves

1 teaspoon sea salt

½ teaspoon black peppercorns

1. Mix all the ingredients together in a large stockpot.

2. Put the pot over high heat and bring the stock to a boil. Reduce the heat, and simmer the stock for 2 hours.

3. Strain the stock through a fine-mesh sieve into jars with sealable lids. Discard the solids.

4. Let the stock cool to room temperature, then seal the jars and store in the refrigerator for up to 4 days, or in the freezer for 3 months.

INGREDIENT TIP: Next time you prepare vegetables for your recipes, save the carrot ends and peelings, celery greens, onion ends, and herb stems for a flavorful vegetable broth. As long as these trimmings are washed, they are fine additions to your stockpot.

PER SERVING (1 cup) Calories: 34; Carbs: 4g; Glycemic Load: 2; Fiber: 0g; Protein: 0g; Sodium: 124mg; Fat: 0g

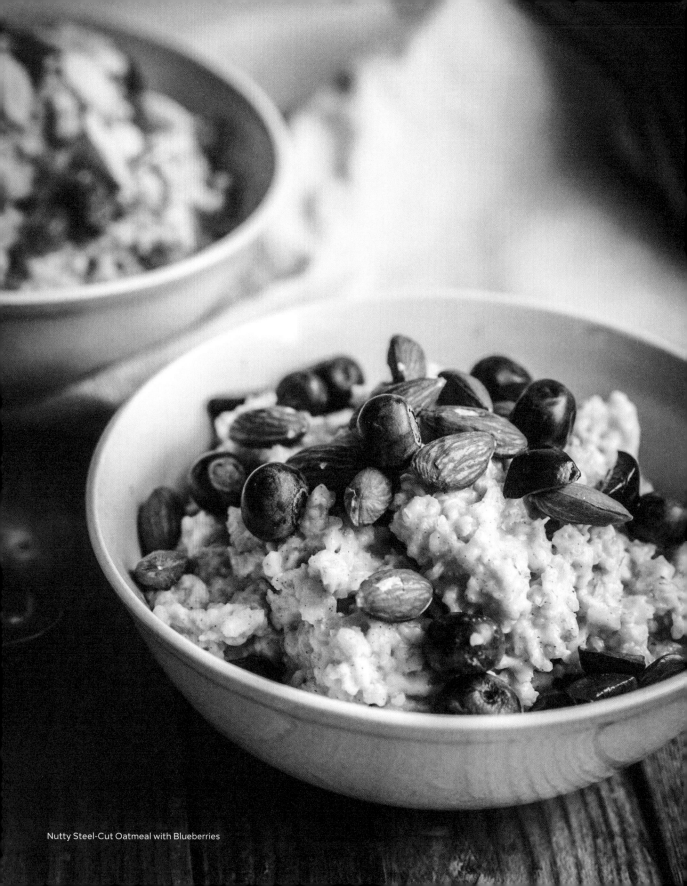

Nutty Steel-Cut Oatmeal with Blueberries

CHAPTER FIVE

Breakfast

NUTTY STEEL-CUT OATMEAL
with Blueberries

PREP TIME: 5 MINUTES · COOK TIME: 30 MINUTES
SERVES 4

Though this oatmeal is delicious on its own, don't forget the blueberry topping, because these sweet berries contain beneficial properties for those with insulin resistance. The phytonutrients in blueberries can reduce the risk of unhealthy belly fat as well as improve insulin sensitivity and glucose levels. Both cultivated and wild blueberries are good choices for your diet.

3 cups water

1 cup steel-cut oats

3 tablespoons almond butter

1 teaspoon ground cinnamon

½ teaspoon ground nutmeg

Pinch ground ginger

1 cup blueberries

½ cup whole almonds

1. Put the water in a medium saucepan over high heat, and bring the liquid to a boil.

2. Stir in the oats, and reduce the heat to low so they simmer gently.

3. Simmer the oats uncovered for about 20 minutes, until they are tender.

4. Stir in the almond butter, cinnamon, nutmeg, and ginger, and simmer for an additional 10 minutes.

5. Serve topped with blueberries and whole almonds.

INGREDIENT TIP: Blueberries can be damaged when shipped, so shake the container gently to see if the berries move freely. Solid sections could indicate crushed berries, or mold. If the blueberries are in a plastic container, turn it upside down to see the ones on the bottom.

PER SERVING Calories: 246; Carbs: 24g; Glycemic Load: 17; Fiber: 5g; Protein: 8g; Sodium: 2mg; Fat: 14g

PEAR-QUINOA HOT CEREAL

PREP TIME: 10 MINUTES • COOK TIME: 15 MINUTES
SERVES 4

You will get a double dose of almonds when sitting down to a steaming bowl of pear-quinoa cereal. Nuts such as almonds are high in fiber, protein, and healthy unsaturated fats, all of which have a positive impact on blood sugar. But be aware that they are also quite high in calories, so consume them in moderation.

1 cup quinoa, rinsed

2 cups unsweetened almond milk, plus extra for serving

1 teaspoon pure vanilla extract

½ teaspoon ground cinnamon

¼ teaspoon ground nutmeg

Pinch ground ginger

2 pears, cored and grated

1 cup slivered almonds

1. Stir together the quinoa, almond milk, vanilla, cinnamon, nutmeg, and ginger in a medium saucepan, and put it on medium heat, covered.

2. Bring the mixture to a simmer, stirring occasionally, then reduce the heat to low and continue to simmer for about 15 minutes, until the quinoa has soaked up most of the liquid.

3. Remove the cereal from the heat, and stir in the pear and almonds.

4. Serve with a drizzle of almond milk.

INGREDIENT TIP: Rinsing quinoa is an important step, because it removes a soapy coating from the seeds called saponins, which can cause digestive problems for some people.

PER SERVING Calories: 379; Carbs: 50g; Glycemic Load: 18; Fiber: 10g; Protein: 12g; Sodium: 94mg; Fat: 16g

5

BAKED OATMEAL CASSEROLE

PREP TIME: 5 MINUTES • COOK TIME: 30 MINUTES
SERVES 4

Oatmeal gets a bad reputation because the market is filled with so many sugar-packed versions that people forget that plain oatmeal is a fabulous start to the day. Oatmeal is a healthy carbohydrate that digests slowly so it doesn't create a spike in blood sugar, just steady energy throughout the morning.

1 teaspoon coconut oil, for greasing the baking dish

1½ cups rolled oats

1 teaspoon baking powder

Pinch sea salt

1¾ cups unsweetened coconut milk (from a carton)

1 tablespoon honey

1 teaspoon pure vanilla extract

¼ teaspoon pure almond extract

¼ cup sunflower seeds

1. Preheat the oven to 375°F.

2. Lightly oil an 8-by-8-inch baking dish and set aside.

3. In a large bowl, stir together the oats, baking powder, and salt.

4. Whisk together the coconut milk, honey, vanilla, almond extract, and sunflower seeds.

5. Add the milk mixture to the oat mixture, and stir to blend.

6. Spoon the oatmeal mixture into the prepared baking dish, and bake for about 30 minutes, until the casserole is golden brown.

7. Serve warm.

COOKING TIP: To save time in the morning, this entire dish can be prepped the evening before and then popped straight into a preheated oven from the refrigerator. Simply increase the cooking time to 45 minutes to offset the chilled ingredients.

PER SERVING Calories: 185; Carbs: 27g; Glycemic Load: 13; Fiber: 3g; Protein: 5g; Sodium: 132mg; Fat: 7g

TOASTY OATMEAL PANCAKES

PREP TIME: 10 MINUTES PLUS 2 HOURS SOAKING TIME • COOK TIME: 21 MINUTES

SERVES 4

There are days when you just need to curl up in your pajamas, and there's nothing like a golden stack of pancakes for some decadent comfort. The batter can be whipped up the night before, and you can just give it a stir in the morning. Whenever possible, use a nutmeg seed and a micrograter to obtain the most intense flavor from the spice.

2 cups rolled oats

2 cups unsweetened almond milk

½ cup almond flour

1 teaspoon baking soda

1 teaspoon baking powder

½ teaspoon ground cinnamon

½ teaspoon ground nutmeg

Pinch sea salt

2 eggs, at room temperature, beaten

¼ cup melted coconut oil, plus extra for cooking

1 teaspoon pure vanilla extract

SERVING TIP: Fresh berries, a dollop of plain yogurt, sliced peaches, or a spoonful of applesauce can all enhance these golden pancakes. You can also store leftover pancakes in the refrigerator and enjoy them cold with a layer of almond butter.

1. Mix the oats and almond milk in a large bowl, and set aside for at least 2 hours (up to overnight) to soften the oats.

2. When you are ready to make the pancakes, in a small bowl, stir together the almond flour, baking soda, baking powder, cinnamon, nutmeg, and salt.

3. Whisk the eggs, melted oil, and vanilla into the oat mixture until blended.

4. Stir the dry ingredients into the wet ingredients until just mixed.

5. Put a large skillet over medium heat, and brush the skillet with oil.

6. Pour the batter into the skillet, ¼ cup per pancake, and cook for about 4 minutes, until the edges are firm and the bottoms golden.

7. Flip the pancakes, and cook for about 3 minutes, until the second side is golden and the pancake is cooked through.

8. Repeat with the remaining batter. Serve 3 pancakes per person.

PER SERVING Calories: 353; Carbs: 31g; Glycemic Load: 15; Fiber: 5g; Protein: 9g; Sodium: 499mg; Fat: 23g

QUINOA WAFFLES

PREP TIME: 10 MINUTES • COOK TIME: 20 MINUTES
SERVES 4

A waffle iron is a good investment for these crispy golden beauties alone. Cinnamon is the main flavoring here, creating a warm, homey fragrance. It is also an excellent addition to your diet if you are trying to manage your blood sugar, because it can significantly lower fasting blood glucose levels.

2 cups unsweetened coconut milk (from a carton)

¼ cup unsweetened applesauce

3 eggs

1½ cups quinoa flour

½ cup almond flour

1 teaspoon baking powder

2 teaspoons ground cinnamon

Pinch ground ginger

Pinch sea salt

1 tablespoon coconut oil, melted

1. Preheat your waffle maker to medium heat.

2. In a small bowl, whisk together the coconut milk, applesauce, and eggs until well blended.

3. In a large bowl, stir together the quinoa flour, almond flour, baking powder, cinnamon, ginger, and salt.

4. Add the wet ingredients to the dry ingredients, and whisk to blend.

5. Brush the waffle iron with coconut oil, and pour ¼ cup of batter into the iron.

6. Cook according to the waffle iron instructions.

7. Repeat with the remaining batter. Serve 2 waffles per person.

COOKING TIP: If you do not have a waffle iron, this batter can also be made into pretty pancakes. Brush a large skillet with coconut oil, and cook them in batches on medium heat.

PER SERVING Calories: 296; Carbs: 15g; Glycemic Load: 19; Fiber: 1g; Protein: 20g; Sodium: 296mg; Fat: 15g

5

TENDER ALMOND PANCAKES

PREP TIME: 5 MINUTES · COOK TIME: 15 MINUTES
SERVES 4

These pancakes can be tricky because the batter is a little delicate, but the end result is worth it. Keep the pancakes small, and use a spatula for flipping that fits under the whole surface. The pancakes will hold together better after they are flipped. Nutmeg, a delicious presence here, can also help decrease blood glucose levels.

2 cups almond flour

2 teaspoons baking powder

1 teaspoon ground cinnamon

¼ teaspoon ground nutmeg

1 cup unsweetened almond milk

4 eggs

1 teaspoon pure vanilla extract

2 tablespoons coconut oil, as needed

INGREDIENT TIP: Almond flour is the almost the same as almond meal, just finer in texture. You can make your own almond flour in a food processor as long as you are careful—don't create almond meal instead by accidentally processing the nuts for too long.

1. In a large bowl, stir together the almond flour, baking powder, cinnamon, and nutmeg.

2. In a small bowl, whisk together the almond milk, eggs, and vanilla.

3. Add the liquid to the almond flour mixture. Stir the batter until just combined.

4. Put a large skillet over medium-high heat, and add 1 tablespoon of coconut oil. When the oil is melted, swirl to coat the skillet.

5. Pour about ¼ cup of batter into the skillet per pancake; you should get 4 pancakes.

6. Cook for about 3 minutes, until bubbles begin to form on the pancakes, then carefully flip them over.

7. Cook on the other side for about 2 minutes, until the pancakes are golden brown.

8. Remove the cooked pancakes to a plate, and cover them with a clean cloth.

9. Repeat with the remaining batter. Serve 3 pancakes per person.

PER SERVING Calories: 228; Carbs: 6g; Glycemic Load: 0; Fiber: 2g; Protein: 10g; Sodium: 122mg; Fat: 20g

TOMATO-HERB OMELET

PREP TIME: 10 MINUTES • COOK TIME: 10 MINUTES
SERVES 2

Herbs can be effective for lowering blood sugar and improving other factors that contribute to insulin action. Fragrant oregano is high in antioxidants that fight free radicals in the body and have a positive effect on an enzyme that breaks down starch into sugar. Including oregano in your recipes can be an effective blood sugar management strategy.

1 tablespoon coconut oil, divided

2 scallions, green and white parts, chopped

1 teaspoon minced garlic

2 tomatoes, chopped, liquid squeezed out

6 eggs, beaten

½ teaspoon chopped fresh thyme

½ teaspoon chopped fresh basil

½ teaspoon chopped fresh chives

½ teaspoon chopped fresh oregano

⅛ teaspoon sea salt

Pinch ground nutmeg

Pinch freshly ground black pepper

Chopped fresh parsley, for garnish

1. Put a small saucepan over medium heat, and add 1 teaspoon of coconut oil.

2. Sauté the scallions and garlic for about 3 minutes, until the vegetables are softened.

3. Add the tomatoes and sauté for 3 minutes. Remove the saucepan from the heat and set aside.

4. In a medium bowl, whisk together the eggs, thyme, basil, chives, oregano, salt, nutmeg, and pepper.

5. Put a large skillet over medium-high heat and add the remaining 2 teaspoons of oil. Swirl the oil until it coats the skillet.

6. Pour in the egg mixture, and swirl until the eggs start to firm up—do not stir the eggs. Lift the edges of the firmed eggs to let the uncooked egg flow underneath.

7. When the eggs are almost set, after about 3 minutes, spoon the tomato mixture onto one-half of the eggs.

8. Fold the uncovered side over the tomato mixture and cook for a minute longer.

9. Cut the omelet in half, sprinkle with parsley, and serve.

INGREDIENT TIP: Any combination of fresh herbs works in this recipe, so give your creative impulses a chance to experiment. Cilantro, savory, marjoram, and dill would all be delicious combined with the other ingredients here.

PER SERVING Calories: 306; Carbs: 13g; Glycemic Load: 3; Fiber: 6g; Protein: 19g; Sodium: 312mg; Fat: 21g

5

VEGETABLE BAKED EGGS

PREP: 15 MINUTES • COOK: 35 MINUTES
SERVES 4

Nature's perfect package for a nutritious meal, eggs are high in protein and unsaturated fat, which keeps you feeling full longer so you won't binge later in the morning. Eggs don't affect blood sugar at all, so try to include them in your diet several times a week—even as a snack, if you like them hardboiled.

2 teaspoons olive oil

1 sweet onion, chopped

2 teaspoons minced garlic

½ small eggplant, diced

1 red bell pepper, seeded and diced

1 yellow bell pepper, seeded and diced

1 zucchini, diced

4 tomatoes, diced

½ cup sodium-free vegetable or chicken broth

1 tablespoon balsamic vinegar

2 tablespoons chopped fresh basil

1 tablespoon chopped fresh oregano

⅛ teaspoon red pepper flakes

4 large eggs

Sea salt

Freshly ground black pepper

1. Put a large skillet over medium-high heat and add the oil.

2. Sauté the onion and garlic for about 4 minutes, until translucent.

3. Add the eggplant and sauté for 5 minutes, until it starts to soften.

4. Add the peppers and zucchini and sauté for 4 minutes.

5. Stir in the tomatoes, stock, and vinegar, and bring the mixture to a boil.

6. Reduce the heat to low and simmer the vegetables for about 20 minutes, stirring occasionally, until they are tender and the liquid is almost completely evaporated.

7. Stir in the basil, oregano, and red pepper flakes.

8. Use the back of a spoon to make 4 deep wells in the vegetable mixture.

9. Crack the eggs into the wells, taking care not to break the yolks.

10. Cover the skillet and let the eggs poach until the whites are firm, about 5 minutes.

11. Serve the eggs with scoops of vegetables, and season with salt and freshly ground black pepper.

INGREDIENT TIP: Eggplant is best when firm, blemish free, and capped with a bright green stem. Make sure you do not cut your eggplant before you use it in the recipe, because this vegetable is extremely perishable and the flesh will discolor.

PER SERVING Calories: 173; Carbs: 18g; Glycemic Load: 6; Fiber: 6g; Protein: 10g; Sodium: 240mg; Fat: 8g

5

ASPARAGUS-SCALLION FRITTATA

PREP TIME: 10 MINUTES • COOK TIME: 18 MINUTES
SERVES 4

The slender, elegant stalks of asparagus in this lovely, simple frittata are a powerful weapon against fluctuating blood sugar levels. Eating asparagus regularly can help suppress your daily blood sugar levels and increase insulin production in the body. Try doubling up on this recipe and eating the frittata cold, wrapped in a multigrain tortilla, for lunch.

8 large eggs

½ cup unsweetened almond milk

1 teaspoon chopped fresh thyme

⅛ teaspoon freshly ground black pepper

Pinch sea salt

2 tablespoons coconut oil

1 teaspoon minced garlic

½ pound asparagus, woody ends trimmed, cut into 2-inch pieces

2 scallions, green and white parts, chopped

½ red bell pepper, finely chopped

INGREDIENT TIP: Asparagus spears should be stored in the supermarket with their ends in shallow water to ensure freshness. When choosing asparagus, keep in mind that any width greater than about a pencil will be woody. Look for tightly closed tips that are slightly deeper green or purplish in color.

1. Preheat the oven to broil.

2. In a medium bowl, whisk together the eggs, almond milk, thyme, pepper, and salt. Set aside.

3. Put a large ovenproof skillet over medium heat, and melt the coconut oil, swirling to coat the sides and bottom.

4. Sauté the garlic until tender, about 3 minutes.

5. Add the asparagus, scallions, and red pepper, and sauté for about 3 minutes, until the vegetables are tender-crisp.

6. Pour the egg mixture into the skillet and cook without agitating the eggs until the edges are set and slightly golden, 7 to 8 minutes.

7. Put the frittata into the preheated oven, and broil for about 4 minutes, until the frittata is golden brown and puffy.

8. Remove the frittata from the oven, and serve.

PER SERVING Calories: 214; Carbs: 5g; Glycemic Load: 2; Fiber: 2g; Protein: 14g; Sodium; 243mg; Fat: 16g

SPINACH AND EGGS SKILLET

PREP TIME: 15 MINUTES • COOK TIME: 20 MINUTES
SERVES 4

Spinach is one of the most nutritious foods you can include in your diet, and this simple breakfast provides a heap of it. Spinach is high in fiber, folate, magnesium, and iron, but it is also considered a "free" food when considering blood sugar impact. Spinach doesn't affect blood sugar levels at all, so eat as much as you like!

1 tablespoon olive oil

1 leek, white and green parts, chopped and washed thoroughly

2 teaspoons minced garlic

10 cups fresh spinach, about 10 ounces

2 teaspoons freshly squeezed lemon juice

4 large eggs

Sea salt

Freshly ground black pepper

1 teaspoon chopped fresh oregano

1. Preheat the oven to 350°F.

2. Put a large skillet over medium heat and add the oil.

3. Sauté the leek and garlic for about 6 minutes, until the vegetables are softened.

4. Add the spinach and lemon juice and sauté for about 4 minutes, tossing with tongs, until the spinach is wilted.

5. Break the eggs onto the spinach, and bake in the oven until the whites are set, about 10 minutes.

6. Remove the skillet from the oven, and season with salt and pepper.

7. Serve sprinkled with oregano.

INGREDIENT TIP: Leeks can be incredibly dirty, so fill up a sink with water, and wash the cut leeks thoroughly by rubbing the pieces between your fingers. Let the leeks float to the surface and the dirt sink to the bottom to ensure that your meal isn't gritty.

PER SERVING Calories: 219; Carbs: 5g; Glycemic Load: 4; Fiber: 2g; Protein: 14g; Sodium: 265mg; Fat: 16g

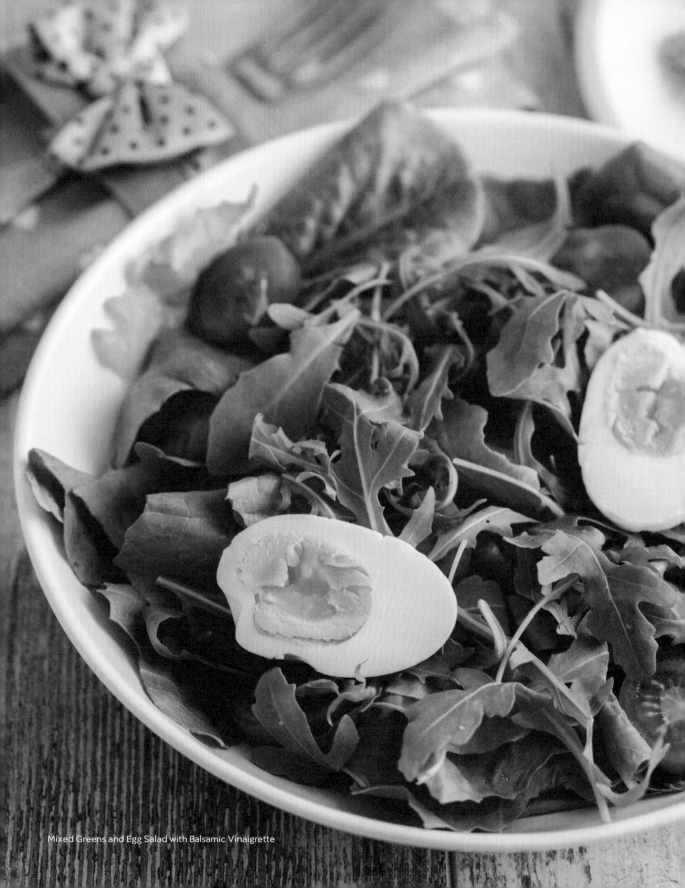

Mixed Greens and Egg Salad with Balsamic Vinaigrette

Salads and Soups

MEDITERRANEAN QUINOA SALAD

PREP TIME: 20 MINUTES
SERVES 4

Quinoa has a high glycemic index, 53, but 4 ounces of this cooked pseudograin has a glycemic load of only 10, and it doesn't cause the blood sugar spikes you might see in potatoes or corn. Quinoa is a complete protein, meaning it contains all the essential amino acids, and it's high in iron and fiber, too.

FOR THE VINAIGRETTE

2 tablespoons apple cider vinegar

2 tablespoons freshly squeezed lemon juice

1 teaspoon Dijon mustard

2 tablespoons chopped fresh oregano

½ cup olive oil

Sea salt

Freshly ground black pepper

FOR THE SALAD

2 cups cooked quinoa

2 tomatoes, diced

2 scallions, white and green parts, chopped

1 red bell pepper, seeded and diced

1 yellow bell pepper, seeded and diced

½ English cucumber, diced

2 tablespoons chopped fresh parsley

TO MAKE THE VINAIGRETTE

1. In a small bowl, whisk the vinegar, lemon juice, Dijon mustard, and oregano until well blended.

2. Whisk in the olive oil, and season with salt and freshly ground black pepper.

TO MAKE THE SALAD

1. In a large bowl, stir together the quinoa, tomatoes, scallions, peppers, and cucumber.

2. Add the vinaigrette to the bowl, and toss until well coated.

3. Sprinkle the salad with parsley, and serve.

SERVING TIP: Serve this salad warm or chilled as a colorful side dish with baked chicken or a perfectly grilled piece of fish. If you prefer it warm, toss the dressing with the hot quinoa and let it sit for 10 to 15 minutes to allow the flavors to fully permeate the dish.

PER SERVING Calories: 422; Carbs: 37g; Glycemic Load: 19; Fiber: 7g; Protein: 8g; Sodium: 86mg; Fat: 39g

6

SUMMER FRUIT AND GREENS SALAD

PREP TIME: 20 MINUTES

SERVES 4

Melon is succulent and exquisitely colored, and bursts with flavor. You can certainly make this salad in winter, but summer-ripe melons will elevate the taste and presentation to sublime. Melon is packed with antioxidants such as beta-carotene, which can boost the immune system and protect you from many diseases, including cardiovascular issues and type 2 diabetes.

FOR THE DRESSING

2 tablespoons apple cider vinegar

1 teaspoon chopped fresh basil

2 tablespoons olive oil

Sea salt

Freshly ground black pepper

FOR THE SALAD

5 cups watercress

2 cups diced watermelon

2 cups diced cantaloupe

½ English cucumber, diced

5 radishes, quartered

1 scallion, white and green parts, chopped

2 tablespoons pumpkin seeds, for garnish

TO MAKE THE DRESSING

1. In a large bowl, whisk together the vinegar, basil, and olive oil until emulsified.

2. Season the vinaigrette with salt and freshly ground black pepper.

TO MAKE THE SALAD

1. Add the watercress to the bowl with the vinaigrette and toss to coat the greens.

2. In a medium bowl, toss together the watermelon, cantaloupe, cucumber, radishes, and scallion.

3. Place the dressed watercress on 4 plates, and top each salad equally with the melon mixture. Garnish with the pumpkin seeds and serve.

INGREDIENT TIP: Watercress is an herb that grows in water, not a lettuce. This peppery perennial is considered one of the most nutrient-dense foods and is best purchased cultivated to avoid the parasites that can be found on wild produce.

PER SERVING Calories: 151; Carbs: 15g; Glycemic Load: 5; Fiber: 2g; Protein: 4g; Sodium: 103mg; Fat: 10g

WHEAT BERRY–GRAPE SALAD

PREP TIME: 30 MINUTES • COOK TIME: 45 MINUTES
SERVES 4

Salads don't have to be an insubstantial mini course or starter—make them a full meal like this one. Wheat berries can be cooked several days in advance and stored in the refrigerator for salads, hot cereals, or as an ingredient in soups. Wheat berries, like other whole grains, are high in fiber and can slow digestion to prevent sugar from flooding into the blood and producing other complications.

FOR THE DRESSING

¼ cup olive oil

2 tablespoons apple cider vinegar

1 tablespoon freshly squeezed lime juice

1 teaspoon honey

1 teaspoon grated fresh ginger

½ teaspoon chopped fresh thyme

Sea salt

FOR THE SALAD

1 cup wheat berries

3 cups water

3 celery stalks, diced

2 cups halved green grapes

1 red apple, cored and chopped

1 scallion, white and green parts, chopped

½ cup chopped fresh mint

½ cup sunflower seeds

6

TO MAKE THE DRESSING

1. In a small bowl, whisk together the olive oil, vinegar, lime juice, honey, ginger, and thyme until emulsified.

2. Season the dressing with salt and set aside.

TO MAKE THE SALAD

1. Put the wheat berries and water in a medium saucepan, and put over high heat.

2. Bring to a boil, then reduce the heat to low and simmer for about 45 minutes, until tender.

3. Drain the wheat berries and transfer them to a large bowl.

4. Let the wheat berries cool for about 30 minutes, and then stir in the celery, grapes, apple, scallion, mint, and sunflower seeds.

5. Add the dressing and toss to coat.

6. Put the salad in the refrigerator, and chill it completely before serving.

SUBSTITUTION TIP: This salad is delicious with quinoa instead of wheat berries if you need to consider a wheat allergy. Increase the quinoa to 1½ cups, and cook with the water until all the liquid is absorbed.

PER SERVING Calories: 296; Carbs: 38g; Glycemic Load: 20; Fiber: 4g; Protein: 4g; Sodium: 86mg; Fat: 16g

QUINOA-LEMON SALAD

PREP TIME: 20 MINUTES

SERVES 4

Kale has an earthy flavor and pleasing crisp texture that holds its own in this attractive salad. Extremely high in vitamins A, C, and K as well as calcium and fiber, kale also contains bile acid sequestrants, which can limit the absorption of dietary fat and help you maintain a healthy weight.

2 cups cooked quinoa

1 cup halved cherry tomatoes

2 cups shredded kale

½ cup slivered almonds

2 tablespoons freshly squeezed lemon juice

1 tablespoon olive oil

Zest of 1 lemon

Sea salt

Freshly ground black pepper

1 avocado, peeled, pitted, and chopped

1. In a large bowl, stir together the quinoa, cherry tomatoes, kale, almonds, lemon juice, olive oil, and lemon zest until well combined.

2. Season the salad with salt and freshly ground black pepper.

3. Top the salad with avocado, and serve.

SUBSTITUTION TIP: In case of a tree nut allergy, exclude the slivered almonds from the dish, and replace with sunflower seeds or pumpkin seeds, which will work equally well for the desired crunch.

PER SERVING Calories: 396; Carbs: 42g; Glycemic Load: 17; Fiber: 9g; Protein: 12g; Sodium: 90mg; Fat: 22g

6

COLORFUL COLESLAW

PREP TIME: 30 MINUTES, PLUS 2 HOURS MARINATING TIME
SERVES 4

Picnics and potluck dinners are traditionally the home of bland mayonnaise-dressed coleslaw—practically no comparison to this zingy, citrus-infused salad. Made with napa cabbage, a frilly delicate-flavored variant, this zippy slaw's better for you, too. Cruciferous vegetables are rich in fiber and have a high water content, which helps control blood glucose levels.

FOR THE DRESSING

2 tablespoons rice vinegar

2 tablespoons sesame oil

1 tablespoon freshly squeezed lime juice

1 teaspoon orange zest

1 teaspoon grated fresh ginger

½ teaspoon minced garlic

FOR THE SALAD

½ head napa cabbage, finely shredded

1 carrot, shredded

2 cups julienned snow peas

2 shallots, chopped

½ cup julienned daikon radish

2 tablespoons chopped fresh cilantro

¼ cup slivered almonds

TO MAKE THE DRESSING

In a small bowl, whisk together the vinegar, sesame oil, lime juice, orange zest, ginger, and garlic. Set aside.

TO MAKE THE SALAD

1. In a large bowl, toss together the cabbage, carrot, snow peas, shallots, radish, cilantro, and almonds.

2. Add the dressing and toss until well coated.

3. Refrigerate the salad for at least 2 hours to intensify the flavor before serving.

> **SUBSTITUTION TIP:** Daikon radish looks a like a fat white carrot with thinner skin. It's milder than regular red radishes, but you can use them if daikon is not available.

PER SERVING Calories: 151; Carbs: 12g; Glycemic Load: 3; Fiber: 4g; Protein: 5g; Sodium: 83mg; Fat: 10g

FRUITED BEAN SALAD

PREP TIME: 15 MINUTES
SERVES 4

Sometimes after a stressful day the last thing you want to do is think about what to eat or deal with a heap of ingredients. This salad keeps in the refrigerator for several days, getting tastier all the time, so you can just come home and enjoy these healthy fiber-packed beans and vegetables right from the container.

2 cups green beans, cut into 1-inch pieces and blanched until tender

1 cup canned navy beans, rinsed well and drained

1 cup canned chickpeas, rinsed well and drained

1 cup canned red kidney beans, rinsed well and drained

1 peach, pitted and finely diced

½ red bell pepper, finely diced

1 scallion, white and green parts, chopped

¼ cup chopped fresh cilantro

2 tablespoons freshly squeezed lime juice

Sea salt

Freshly ground black pepper

1. In a large bowl, stir together the green beans, navy beans, chickpeas, red kidney beans, peach, red pepper, scallion, cilantro, and lime juice.

2. Season the salad with salt and freshly ground black pepper, and serve.

COOKING TIP: Blanching vegetables is simple, but too much time in boiling water can produce a mushy texture. The trick to al dente green beans is to have a large bowl filled with ice and cold water ready: Plunge the blanched drained beans into the ice water to arrest the cooking process.

PER SERVING Calories: 195; Carbs: 36g; Glycemic Load: 18; Fiber: 12g; Protein: 11g; Sodium: 272mg; Fat: 2g

MIXED GREENS AND EGG SALAD
with Balsamic Vinaigrette

PREP TIME: 20 MINUTES
SERVES 4

Tomatoes are sweet and pop with vibrant color in salads and other dishes—they are also high in vitamins C and E as well as iron. For a truly sublime taste, source out heirloom tomatoes in different colors, and cut them into the salad at room temperature when their flavor is strongest.

FOR THE DRESSING

3 tablespoons white balsamic vinegar

1 teaspoon chopped fresh tarragon

5 tablespoons olive oil

Sea salt

Freshly ground black pepper

FOR THE SALAD

6 cups mixed baby greens

2 cups halved cherry tomatoes

4 hardboiled eggs, cut in half lengthwise

½ red onion, thinly sliced (optional)

TO MAKE THE DRESSING

1. In a small bowl, whisk together the vinegar, tarragon, and olive oil.

2. Season the dressing with salt and freshly ground black pepper.

TO MAKE THE SALAD

1. In a large bowl, toss the mixed baby greens together with half of the dressing.

2. Arrange the salad on 4 plates.

3. Top each salad with ½ cup cherry tomatoes and 2 hardboiled egg halves.

4. Drizzle the remaining dressing on the salads, and serve topped with sliced red onion (if using).

SUBSTITUTION TIP: Omitting the egg creates a dish suitable for vegans. If you want to add more protein to the dish, top each salad with a couple of tablespoons of toasted sunflower seeds.

PER SERVING Calories: 285; Carbs: 15g; Glycemic Load: 2; Fiber: 6g; Protein: 11g; Sodium: 184mg; Fat: 22g

ARUGULA CHICKEN SALAD
with Tahini Dressing

PREP TIME: 15 MINUTES
SERVES 4

Lean cooked chicken can be used in salads, soups, and snacks to add extra protein and nutrients to your meals. Grass-fed organic chicken tastes better than commercially raised birds, and has a better nutrition profile, with less saturated fat as well as higher levels of omega-3 fatty acids and vitamin A.

FOR THE DRESSING

½ cup freshly squeezed lime juice

2 tablespoons tahini

1 teaspoon honey

¼ teaspoon minced garlic

¼ cup olive oil

FOR THE SALAD

4 cups arugula

1 cup baby spinach

2 cups snap peas, stringed and cut in half crosswise

1 cup 1-inch asparagus, pieces

1 scallion, white and green parts, chopped

3 cups diced cooked chicken

TO MAKE THE DRESSING

1. In a small bowl, whisk together the lime juice, tahini, honey, and garlic.

2. Whisk in the olive oil until the dressing is blended, and set aside.

TO MAKE THE SALAD

1. In a large bowl, toss together the arugula, spinach, snap peas, asparagus, and scallion until mixed. Add three-quarters of the dressing, and toss to coat the ingredients.

2. Arrange the salad on 4 plates, and top evenly with the cooked chicken.

3. Drizzle the remaining dressing evenly over the salads, and serve.

INGREDIENT TIP: Cooking batches of chicken breasts at the beginning of the week and storing them in sealed plastic bags in the refrigerator can save time with recipes such as this salad. Chicken will keep for up to 5 days if chilled completely and wrapped properly.

PER SERVING Calories: 398; Carbs: 17g; Glycemic Load: 3; Fiber: 6g; Protein: 37g; Sodium: 91mg; Fat: 20g

SPICY VEGETABLE SOUP

PREP TIME: 25 MINUTES • COOK TIME: 45 MINUTES
SERVES 4

Fiber, flavor, and fabulous colors are combined in one bowl in this bountiful vegetable soup. Don't throw out the celery greens—chop them up to add to the taste of the broth. Celery is another excellent food for stabilizing your blood sugar: The fiber in celery turns into a jellylike substance during digestion that dramatically slows the absorption of sugar, producing more balanced blood glucose levels.

2 tablespoons olive oil

1 sweet onion, chopped

2 teaspoons minced garlic

2 carrots, cut in half crosswise

2 celery stalks, chopped

½ fennel bulb, chopped

2 cups shredded green cabbage

1 sweet potato, peeled and diced

8 cups low-sodium chicken broth

2 teaspoons chopped fresh thyme

¼ teaspoon chili powder

Pinch red pepper flakes

1 cup shredded kale

Sea salt

Freshly ground black pepper

1. Put a large stockpot over medium-high heat, and add the olive oil.

2. Add the onion and minced garlic to the stockpot, and sauté for about 4 minutes, until the vegetables are tender.

3. Add the carrot, celery, fennel, cabbage, and sweet potato to the pot, and sauté for 5 minutes, stirring constantly.

4. Stir in the chicken broth, thyme, chili powder, and red pepper flakes.

5. Bring the soup to a boil, then reduce the heat to low and simmer for about 30 minutes, until the vegetables are tender.

6. Stir in the kale, and simmer for 4 minutes.

7. Season the soup with salt and freshly ground black pepper, and serve.

INGREDIENT TIP: Fennel has a delightful licorice flavor that combines beautifully with the thyme. For an extra-special taste, chop the feathery fennel greens into the soup as well.

PER SERVING Calories: 171; Carbs: 21g; Glycemic Load: 7; Fiber: 5g; Protein: 7g; Sodium: 269mg; Fat: 7g

SPRING ASPARAGUS AND SNAP PEA SOUP

PREP TIME: 20 MINUTES · COOK TIME: 40 MINUTES

SERVES 4

This soup is a perfect choice for elevating your mood. But don't cook the asparagus and snap peas too long: These vegetables should still be slightly crisp when you remove the soup from the heat to purée it, or you won't get that happy bright green you hoped for.

1 teaspoon olive oil

1 leek, white and green parts, chopped and cleaned well

1 teaspoon minced garlic

6 cups sodium-free vegetable broth

½ cup brown rice

1 pound asparagus, woody ends trimmed, cut into 1-inch pieces

½ pound snap peas

2 tablespoons freshly squeezed lemon juice

1 tablespoon chopped fresh thyme

Pinch ground nutmeg

Sea salt

Freshly ground black pepper

SERVING TIP: This soup is gloriously green and has a subtle lemon undertone. If you need a special meal on hot summer days, chill this soup and serve it topped with pink chive flowers.

1. Put a large stockpot over medium heat, and add the olive oil.

2. Sauté the leek and garlic in the oil for about 5 minutes, until the vegetables are softened.

3. Stir in the vegetable broth and rice, and bring the liquid to a boil.

4. Reduce the heat to low and simmer for about 30 minutes, until the rice is tender.

5. Stir in the asparagus, snap peas, lemon juice, and thyme, and increase the heat to medium so that the soup simmers.

6. Simmer for about 5 minutes, until the vegetables are tender and bright green.

7. Remove the soup from the heat, and transfer it to a food processor.

8. Purée the soup until it is smooth and silky, and stir in the nutmeg.

9. Season the soup with salt and freshly ground black pepper, and serve immediately.

PER SERVING Calories: 206; Carbs: 41g; Glycemic Load: 15; Fiber: 7g; Protein: 8g; Sodium: 116mg; Fat: 2g

CURRIED CAULIFLOWER SOUP

PREP TIME: 20 MINUTES • COOK TIME: 40 MINUTES
SERVES 4

Curry and cauliflower are natural culinary friends, and you will find them side by side in many traditional dishes from India and North Africa. Cumin can reduce fasting blood sugar levels when eaten as a regular part of your diet. Cauliflower purées to a silky-smooth texture when cooked, and the extra blanched florets add back some chunky goodness.

2 heads cauliflower, cut into small florets, divided

½ teaspoon olive oil

1 sweet onion, chopped

2 teaspoons minced garlic

4 cups sodium-free vegetable broth

1 (14-ounce) can coconut milk

2 teaspoons curry powder

1 teaspoon garam masala

½ teaspoon ground cumin

Sea salt

2 tablespoons chopped fresh cilantro

> **INGREDIENT TIP:** Garam masala is a spice blend common in North Indian food, usually composed of cumin, cloves, black peppercorns, nutmeg, and cardamom. You can make your own mix or purchase a premade product at the local grocery store.

1. Put a medium saucepan filled with water over high heat, and bring to a boil.

2. Blanch half of the cauliflower florets for about 3 minutes, until tender, then drain and set aside.

3. Put a large saucepan over medium heat, and add the olive oil.

4. Sauté the onion and garlic for about 4 minutes, until softened.

5. Stir in the remaining cauliflower, broth, coconut milk, curry, garam masala, and cumin.

6. Bring the soup to a boil, then reduce the heat to low and simmer for about 30 minutes, until the cauliflower is tender.

7. Transfer the soup to a food processor, and purée until smooth and creamy.

8. Pour the soup back into the saucepan, and add the blanched cauliflower.

9. Season the soup with salt and freshly ground black pepper.

10. Serve sprinkled with cilantro.

PER SERVING Calories: 288; Carbs: 18g; Glycemic Load: 7; Fiber: 6g; Protein: 5g; Sodium: 146mg; Fat: 24g

NAVY BEAN AND TOMATO SOUP

PREP TIME: 20 MINUTES · COOK TIME: 1 HOUR, 10 MINUTES
SERVES 4

The ingredients listed here are just a suggestion for getting started creating your own hearty meal; the beans and tomatoes are really the only ingredients that should remain constant. Cauliflower, carrots, green beans, kale, and cabbage are all vegetables that would also combine well with the other flavors and textures. Including an assortment of vegetables in your diet will help you meet your fiber and nutrient needs, which helps boost your immunity and reduce blood sugar spikes.

2 tablespoons olive oil

1 sweet onion, diced

2 celery stalks, diced

2 teaspoons minced garlic

2 bay leaves

1 tablespoon chopped fresh thyme

8 cups low-sodium vegetable broth

1 cup dry navy beans, picked through, soaked for 2 hours and drained

1 (4-ounce) can organic tomato paste

2 large tomatoes, diced

1 cup chopped fresh spinach

Sea salt

Freshly ground black pepper

1. Put a large stockpot over medium-high heat and add the olive oil.

2. Sauté the onion, celery, and garlic for 3 to 4 minutes, until softened.

3. Add the bay leaves, thyme, broth, beans, tomato paste, and tomatoes to the pot.

4. Bring the soup to a boil, then reduce the heat to low and simmer the soup for about 1 hour, until the beans are tender.

5. Remove the bay leaves, and stir in the spinach.

6. Simmer for 2 minutes.

7. Season the soup with salt and freshly ground black pepper, and serve.

INGREDIENT TIP: Dried navy beans need to be picked through because rocks and bits of grit can be scooped into the bags during the picking and packaging process. Canned sodium-free navy beans are a good option, too, if you want to save about 30 minutes of cooking time.

PER SERVING Calories: 335; Carbs: 53g; Glycemic Load: 15; Fiber: 18g; Protein: 16g; Sodium: 388mg; Fat: 8g

6

GREEN POWER SOUP

PREP TIME: 15 MINUTES • COOK TIME: 15 MINUTES
SERVES 4

All the vegetables chopped and simmered in this pot are green and packed with nutrients, allowing your body to bask in iron, vitamins A, C, and K, as well as calcium, magnesium, potassium, and multiple antioxidants. Whip up a batch of this soup in the winter months, when your body's immunity and energy are both low.

1 tablespoon olive oil

1 leek, white and light green parts, sliced crosswise and washed thoroughly

2 celery stalks, diced

2 teaspoons minced garlic

6 cups sodium-free chicken broth

2 cups shredded kale

1 cup shredded green cabbage

1 cup green snap peas

1 cup shredded spinach

1 tablespoon chopped fresh basil

1 tablespoon chopped fresh thyme

Juice of 1 lemon

1 teaspoon lemon zest

Sea salt

Freshly ground black pepper

¼ cup pumpkin seeds

1. Put a large stockpot over medium-high heat, and add the olive oil.

2. Sauté the leek, celery, and garlic for about 5 minutes, until softened.

3. Stir in the chicken broth and bring the soup to a boil.

4. Add the kale, cabbage, peas, spinach, basil, and thyme to the pot.

5. Reduce the heat to low and simmer the soup for about 10 minutes, until the vegetables are tender.

6. Stir in the lemon juice and zest, and purée the soup in a food processor until very smooth.

7. Season the soup with salt and freshly ground black pepper.

8. Serve topped with pumpkin seeds.

SUBSTITUTION TIP: Using vegetable broth instead of chicken broth allows your vegan and vegetarian friends to indulge in this nutrient-packed soup. Homemade stock is best, but high-quality organic sodium-free products also serve nicely.

PER SERVING Calories: 170; Carbs: 17g; Glycemic Load: 5; Fiber: 4g; Protein: 9g; Sodium: 220mg; Fat: 8g

CITRUSY SEAFOOD SOUP

PREP TIME: 15 MINUTES • COOK TIME: 15 MINUTES
SERVES 4

This soup contains a generous quantity of grated fresh ginger to enhance the flavor of the seafood. Thought to help prevent several forms of cancer such as ovarian and colon cancer, ginger is also a powerful anti-inflammatory and painkiller that can reduce the severity of migraines, heartburn, inflammation of the joints, and nausea.

1 teaspoon olive oil

2 teaspoons minced garlic

1 teaspoon grated fresh ginger

6 cups sodium-free vegetable broth

½ cup clam juice

2 (6-ounce) firm white fish fillets, cut into 1-inch chunks (haddock, halibut, cod)

6 sea scallops, halved

1 large carrot, finely diced

Juice and zest of 1 lime

2 scallions, white and green parts, thinly sliced

1 red bell pepper, seeded and diced

2 tablespoons chopped fresh cilantro

¼ teaspoon red pepper flakes

1. Put a large stockpot over medium-high heat, and add the oil.

2. Sauté the garlic and ginger for about 3 minutes, until softened.

3. Stir in the broth and clam juice, and bring the soup to a boil.

4. Reduce the heat to low and add the fish, scallops, and carrot.

5. Simmer the soup for about 8 minutes, until the seafood is just cooked through.

6. Stir in the juice, zest, scallions, red pepper, cilantro, and red pepper flakes.

7. Simmer for 1 minute, and serve immediately.

INGREDIENT TIP: Clam juice is probably an ingredient you have walked past countless times in the grocery store without noticing the can or bottle. Look for it in the section with canned tuna, salmon, clams, and sardines.

PER SERVING Calories: 215; Carbs: 9g; Glycemic Load: 2; Fiber: 2g; Protein: 32g; Sodium: 654mg; Fat: 5g

6

CHICKEN BARLEY SOUP

PREP TIME: 10 MINUTES • COOK TIME: 35 MINUTES
SERVES 4

Soup plays a prominent role in many childhoods as the meal that meant comfort and home. This hearty soup can almost be eaten with a fork because it is so thick with vegetables, chunks of tender chicken, and chewy barley. Barley is a tasty whole grain with the same positive effect on the body as other high-fiber foods: slower blood sugar absorption.

2 teaspoons olive oil

1 sweet onion, chopped

3 celery stalks, diced

2 carrots, sliced into thin rounds

8 cups sodium-free chicken broth

½ cup pearl barley

1 tablespoon chopped fresh thyme

3 cups chopped cooked chicken meat

1 cup shredded kale

Sea salt

Freshly ground black pepper

Chopped fresh parsley, for garnish

1. Put a large saucepan over medium-high heat, and add the olive oil.

2. Sauté the onion, celery, and carrot for about 5 minutes, until the vegetables are softened.

3. Stir in the broth, barley, and thyme.

4. Bring the soup to a boil, then reduce the heat to low and simmer for about 20 minutes, until the barley is tender.

5. Stir in the cooked chicken and kale, and simmer for 5 minutes.

6. Season the soup with salt and freshly ground black pepper.

7. Sprinkle with parsley, and serve.

SUBSTITUTION TIP: This recipe can be converted to a vegan or vegetarian meal by leaving out the chicken and using vegetable broth. The abundant vegetables and barley are hearty enough for a light dinner or satisfying lunch.

PER SERVING Calories: 383; Carbs: 32g; Glycemic Load: 14; Fiber: 6g; Protein: 36g; Sodium: 421mg; Fat: 12g

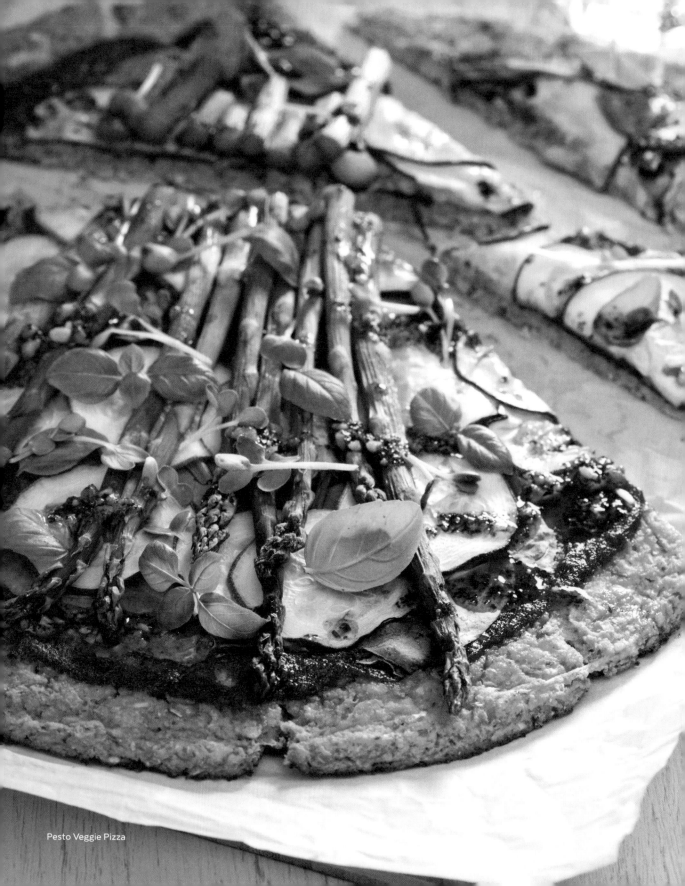
Pesto Veggie Pizza

CHAPTER SEVEN

Snacks and Sides

GUACAMOLE DIP

PREP TIME: 15 MINUTES
SERVES 8

Guacamole is easy to whip up when you need something delicious very quickly. The healthy fat in the avocado can help you feel fuller longer and reduce the urge to overeat. You shouldn't keep guacamole around very long—it can oxidize to an unattractive grayish color. Make sure you stir the guacamole before serving, so the oxidized portion gets blended into the rest.

2 ripe avocados, peeled and pitted

1 tomato, diced

½ jalapeño pepper, finely chopped

2 tablespoons freshly squeezed lime juice

½ teaspoon minced garlic

¼ teaspoon salt

1. In a medium bowl, mash the avocados until smooth. Stir in the tomato, jalapeño pepper, lime juice, garlic, and salt.

2. Store in the refrigerator in a sealed container for up to 2 days.

INGREDIENT TIP: Jalapeño peppers require careful handling because the juices and seeds can burn the mucus membranes of the body. Always wash your hands thoroughly after cutting or handling the peppers, and scrub off any surfaces you've used for cutting them.

PER SERVING Calories: 104; Carbs: 5g; Glycemic Load: 2; Fiber: 3g; Protein: 1g; Sodium: 76mg; Fat: 10g

GARLICKY HUMMUS

PREP TIME: 15 MINUTES
MAKES 2 CUPS

If you are searching for a filling snack, look no further than this nutrition-packed recipe. The main ingredients of hummus are chickpeas and tahini, both of which practically burst with fiber, protein, and unsaturated fats—all blood-sugar-controlling elements. Chickpeas contain almost 12 grams of fiber and over 15 grams of protein per cup, making them a nutritional superstar.

1½ cups canned chickpeas, rinsed and drained

¼ cup tahini

2 teaspoons minced garlic

1 teaspoon ground cumin

½ teaspoon ground coriander

¼ cup freshly squeezed lemon juice

2 tablespoons olive oil

Sea salt

1. Put the chickpeas, tahini, garlic, cumin, coriander, and lemon juice in a food processor, and blend until smooth, scraping down the sides of the processor at least once.

2. Add the olive oil and process until blended. Season with sea salt.

3. Store the hummus in a sealed container in the refrigerator for up to 1 week.

SERVING TIP: Hummus is not just a tasty dip; it can be used in many different applications in your kitchen. This smooth garlicky purée is equally spectacular stirred into sauces, spread on sandwiches, and used as a topping for soups.

PER SERVING (¼ cup) Calories: 147; Carbs: 14g; Glycemic Load: 10; Fiber: 4g; Protein: 5g; Sodium: 35mg; Fat: 9g

PESTO VEGGIE PIZZA

PREP TIME: 20 MINUTES • COOK TIME: 15 MINUTES
SERVES 8

The crust for this healthy snack takes a bit of work to create, but the result is a guilt-free version of the traditional calorie-laden crust. You want about 3 cups of cauliflower "flour"; if you end up with more, set it aside for another recipe. To save time, you can also microwave the ground cauliflower rather than steaming it.

Olive oil, for greasing the parchment paper

1 head cauliflower, cut into florets

3 tablespoons almond flour

2 teaspoons olive oil

1 egg, beaten

½ teaspoon minced garlic

Pinch sea salt

1 cup Simple Tomato Sauce (page 76)

1 zucchini, thinly sliced

1 cup baby spinach leaves

10 asparagus spears, woody ends trimmed, cut into 3-inch pieces

¼ cup basil pesto

1. Preheat the oven to 450°F. Put an unrimmed baking sheet in the oven.

2. Lightly brush a piece of parchment paper with olive oil, and set aside.

3. Put a large saucepan filled halfway with water over high heat, and bring it to a boil.

4. Put the cauliflower in a food processor, and pulse until very finely chopped, almost flour consistency.

5. Transfer the ground cauliflower to a fine-mesh sieve, and put it over the boiling water for about 1 minute, until the cauliflower is cooked.

6. Transfer the cauliflower to a clean kitchen towel, and wring out all the water. Transfer the cauliflower to a large bowl.

7. Stir in the almond flour, oil, egg, garlic, and salt, and mix to create a thick dough. Use your hands to press the ingredients together, and transfer the cauliflower mixture to the parchment paper.

8. Press the mixture out into a flat circle, about ½ inch thick. Slide the parchment paper onto the baking sheet in the oven.

9. Bake the crust for about 10 minutes, until it is crisp and turns golden brown.

10. Remove the crust from the oven, and spread the sauce evenly to the edges of the crust.

11. Arrange the zucchini, spinach, and asparagus on the pizza.

12. Drizzle the pizza with the basil pesto, and put it back in the oven for about 2 minutes, until the vegetables are tender. Serve.

SUBSTITUTION TIP: If the preparation of the cauliflower crust seems like too much work, another option is to use a gluten-free crust. Look for a crust with limited ingredients that doesn't contain any items you are trying to avoid.

PER SERVING Calories: 107; Carbs: 8g; Glycemic Load: 5; Fiber :3g; Protein: 5g; Sodium: 64mg; Fat: 7g

APPLE LEATHER

PREP TIME: 10 MINUTES • COOK TIME: 8 TO 10 HOURS

MAKES 24 STRIPS

You will have moments in the day when the urge to indulge in something sweet will overwhelm you. Instead of snacking on something that will create wildly fluctuating blood sugar, reach for a couple of strips of apple leather. Apples are nutritional powerhouses that can help lower cholesterol and control blood sugar.

5 apples, peeled, cored, and sliced

¼ cup water

1 teaspoon pure vanilla extract

¼ teaspoon ground ginger

¼ teaspoon ground cloves

INGREDIENT TIP: Pears, peaches, and strawberries can also be made into delicious fruit leathers, or, if you are feeling creative, try mixing them. To ensure a smooth result, take the time to strain out the strawberry seeds before spreading the purée on the baking sheet.

1. Put the apples, water, vanilla, ginger, and cloves in a large saucepan over medium heat.

2. Bring the mixture to a boil, reduce the heat to low, and simmer for about 20 minutes, until the apples are very tender.

3. Transfer the apple mixture to a food processor, and purée until very smooth.

4. Set the oven on the lowest possible setting.

5. Line a baking sheet with parchment paper.

6. Pour the puréed apple mixture onto the baking sheet, and spread it out very thinly and evenly.

7. Put the baking sheet in the oven, and bake for 8 to 10 hours, until the leather is smooth and no longer sticky.

8. Cut the apple leather with a pizza cutter into 24 strips, and store this treat in a sealed container in a cool, dark place for up to 2 weeks.

PER SERVING (2 strips) Calories: 41; Carbs: 11g; Glycemic Load: 2; Fiber: 2g; Protein: 0g; Sodium: 1mg; Fat: 0g

SIMPLE APPETIZER MEATBALLS

PREP TIME: 25 MINUTES • COOK TIME: 25 MINUTES
MAKES 24

Meatballs make a charming snack, perfect for guests and family stopping over for a festive visit. A platter of meatballs surrounded by a variety of tasty dips can take the edge off your hunger without filling you up completely. Try these meatballs with a sweet and spicy dipping sauce or a splash of hot pepper sauce.

½ pound lean ground beef

½ pound lean ground pork

½ cup sodium-free chicken broth

¼ cup almond flour

1 tablespoon low-sodium tamari sauce

½ teaspoon ground cumin

¼ teaspoon freshly ground black pepper

1. Preheat the oven to 375°F.

2. In a large bowl, mix all the ingredients together until completely incorporated.

3. Roll the mixture into ¾-inch balls, and place them on a parchment-lined baking sheet.

4. Bake the meatballs for 25 to 30 minutes, until they are cooked through and golden brown. Serve.

COOKING TIP: You can easily freeze these meatballs, raw or cooked, to keep a speedy snack on hand for yourself or guests. If you cook the meatballs first, chill them completely in the refrigerator before transferring to plastic freezer bags.

PER SERVING (4 meatballs) Calories: 125; Carbs: 0g; Glycemic Load: 0; Fiber: 0g; Protein: 20g; Sodium: 157mg; Fat: 4g

SOUTHWESTERN RICE

PREP TIME: 20 MINUTES • COOK TIME: 45 MINUTES
SERVES 6

The sunny color of this side dish comes from turmeric, a traditional spice used extensively in Asian cooking. Turmeric contains a volatile essential oil called curcumin, which acts as a powerful anti-inflammatory. Eating turmeric regularly can decrease blood glucose levels. And while it might seem a little strange at first to add this spice to a Southwestern dish, it complements those flavors beautifully.

1 tablespoon olive oil

½ sweet onion, finely chopped

1 teaspoon minced garlic

1 red bell pepper, seeded and finely chopped

1 green bell pepper, seeded and finely chopped

1 carrot, finely chopped

1 teaspoon ground cumin

1 teaspoon ground coriander

¼ teaspoon ground turmeric

1 cup brown rice

2 cups low-sodium chicken broth

1. Put a large saucepan over medium-high heat, and add the olive oil.

2. Sauté the onion and garlic for about 3 minutes, until the vegetables are softened.

3. Add the peppers, carrot, cumin, coriander, and turmeric to the saucepan.

4. Sauté the vegetables for 5 minutes.

5. Add the brown rice and chicken broth to the saucepan, and stir to combine.

6. Bring the rice to a boil, then reduce the heat and simmer, covered, for about 35 minutes, until the liquid is absorbed.

7. Stir, and serve.

SUBSTITUTION TIP: Swap the chicken broth for a flavorful vegetable broth if you are looking for a vegan or vegetarian side dish. Homemade vegetable stock is simple to make and costs pennies per serving, so try your hand at whipping up your own.

PER SERVING Calories: 162; Carbs: 29g; Glycemic Load: 18; Fiber: 2g; Protein: 4g; Sodium: 34mg; Fat: 3g

GERMAN-STYLE RED CABBAGE

PREP TIME: 10 MINUTES • COOK TIME: 65 MINUTES
SERVES 4

Boiled cabbage cooked on its own can smell pretty unpleasant. This preparation, on the other hand, smells heavenly, featuring sweet pears, tangy apple cider vinegar, and sautéed onion. All the main ingredients in this side dish are low-GI and very high in fiber. As an added bonus, red cabbage braises to a deep ruby red that is gorgeous on any plate.

1 teaspoon olive oil

1 head red cabbage, shredded

1 sweet onion, thinly sliced

2 pears, peeled, cored, and diced

¼ cup apple cider vinegar

¼ teaspoon salt

⅛ teaspoon freshly ground black pepper

1. Put a large saucepan over medium heat, and add the oil.

2. Sauté the cabbage and onion for about 6 minutes, until it softens and starts to purge liquid.

3. Add the pears, apple cider vinegar, salt, and freshly ground black pepper to the saucepan.

4. Cover the pot and reduce the heat to low.

5. Cook the cabbage for about 1 hour, stirring occasionally, until the vegetables are very tender. Serve hot.

COOKING TIP: Braised cabbage is very easy to make in a slow cooker if you just want to set it and forget it. Add ½ cup of water to the pot with the other ingredients, and cook on low for 6 hours.

PER SERVING Calories: 114; Carbs: 32g; Glycemic Load: 8; Fiber: 10g; Protein: 4g; Sodium: 191mg; Fat: 2g

BEANS with Sun-Dried Tomatoes

PREP TIME: 20 MINUTES · COOK TIME: 1 HOUR
SERVES 8

Baked or simmered beans seem to belong over a smoky campfire, cooking in the open air with the scent of pine trees. You can certainly try this recipe under those conditions, but a cozy stovetop at home also works nicely. If you have a slow cooker, prepare the recipe on low for 6 hours.

3 (14-ounce) cans navy beans, rinsed and drained

1 cup low-sodium vegetable broth

2 teaspoons minced garlic

1 cup chopped sun-dried tomatoes

1 teaspoon ground cumin

Sea salt

1. Put the beans, broth, garlic, sun-dried tomatoes, and cumin in a saucepan over medium-high heat.

2. Bring the liquid to a simmer, and reduce the heat to low.

3. Simmer the beans, stirring occasionally, for about 1 hour, until the beans are very tender and the liquid is evaporated.

4. Season with sea salt, and serve.

INGREDIENT TIP: Sun-dried tomatoes are packed with flavor and nutrients but can also be high in fat if you get them packed in oil. Try to find this ingredient in dried form (sold in bags) because you will be simmering them in liquid, which plumps them back up with moisture.

PER SERVING Calories: 272; Carbs: 48g; Glycemic Load: 17; Fiber: 20g; Protein: 18g; Sodium: 186mg; Fat: 1g

ROASTED BRUSSELS SPROUTS
with Walnuts

PREP TIME: 15 MINUTES • COOK TIME: 25 MINUTES

SERVES 4

Roasting vegetables makes them sweeter and imparts a pleasing smoky flavor; Brussels sprouts are no exception, and their high fiber and nutrient content supports the Insulin Resistance Diet. Cut the woody ends off the sprouts and slice a small "X" on the cut edge, to give the less tender part of this vegetable a chance to cook through, while also lending an appetizing look to the dish.

1 pound Brussels sprouts, halved lengthwise

2 tablespoons walnut oil

Sea salt

Freshly ground black pepper

1 teaspoon chopped fresh thyme

¼ cup chopped walnuts

1. Preheat the oven to 400°F.

2. Line a baking sheet with aluminum foil.

3. In a large bowl, toss the Brussels sprouts with the oil and lightly season with salt and freshly ground black pepper.

4. Spread the Brussels sprouts on the baking sheet, and roast for 20 to 25 minutes, stirring at least once, until the vegetables start to brown.

5. Toss the roasted Brussels sprouts with thyme, and serve topped with chopped walnuts.

SUBSTITUTION TIP: The walnut oil and chopped walnuts can be replaced with olive oil and roasted sunflower seeds if your diet does not permit you to eat tree nuts.

PER SERVING Calories: 122; Carbs: 12g; Glycemic Load: 3; Fiber: 5g; Protein: 7g; Sodium: 87mg; Fat: 7g

LEMON ASPARAGUS

PREP TIME: 10 MINUTES • COOK TIME: 6 MINUTES
SERVES 4

Lemon and asparagus have a long history as culinary counterparts—tangy citrus doesn't overpower this delicate green vegetable. Don't overcook your asparagus, or the vegetables will get mushy. This dish is tasty served cold the next day as a snack, or added to a light lunch.

2 pounds asparagus, woody ends trimmed

1 tablespoon olive oil

⅛ teaspoon sea salt

1 tablespoon white balsamic vinegar

2 tablespoons freshly squeezed lemon juice

1 teaspoon lemon zest

2 teaspoons chopped fresh thyme

1. Preheat the oven to 400°F.

2. Line a baking sheet with aluminum foil.

3. In a large bowl, toss together the asparagus, olive oil, and salt.

4. Arrange the asparagus on the baking sheet in a single layer, and roast in the oven for about 6 minutes, until tender and lightly browned.

5. Transfer the asparagus to a bowl, toss with the vinegar, lemon juice, zest, and thyme, and serve.

SUBSTITUTION TIP: White balsamic vinegar can be hard to locate in some stores, but it is worth finding for its mellow sweet flavor. If white balsamic is not available, you can substitute regular balsamic instead, measure for measure.

PER SERVING Calories: 80; Carbs: 9g; Glycemic Load: 1; Fiber: 5g; Protein: 5g; Sodium: 65mg; Fat: 4g

CHILI-ROASTED CHICKPEAS

PREP TIME: 5 MINUTES • COOK TIME: 30 MINUTES
SERVES 6

Sometimes a snack with the combination of crunchy and spicy is exactly what you need to satisfy a craving. These golden beauties have the added bonus of being a fabulous source of fiber and healthy fat. You can adjust the spices to suit your own palate and if you prefer a plainer flavor, omit the seasoning altogether and top with a light sprinkle of sea salt instead.

1 (15-ounce) can chickpeas, drained, rinsed and dried

1 tablespoon olive oil, plus extra for greasing

1 teaspoon chili powder

¼ teaspoon sea salt

Pinch cayenne powder

1. Preheat the oven to 400°F.

2. Place the chickpeas in a medium bowl and add the olive oil, chili powder, salt, and cayenne. Toss to evenly coat the chickpeas with the oil and spices.

3. Transfer the spiced chickpeas to a lightly greased baking sheet and bake until lightly golden and crisp, about 30 minutes. Shake the tray at least once in the middle of this baking process.

4. Cool the chickpeas completely before serving. You can also store them in a sealed container at room temperature for up to 3 days.

COOKING TIP: Make sure you use a baking sheet with at least a ½-inch rim. Otherwise, your chickpeas might roll off when you try to shake them as they bake.

PER SERVING Calories: 107; Carbs: 12g; Glycemic Load: 6; Fiber: 3g; Protein: 5g; Sodium: 90mg; Fat: 5g

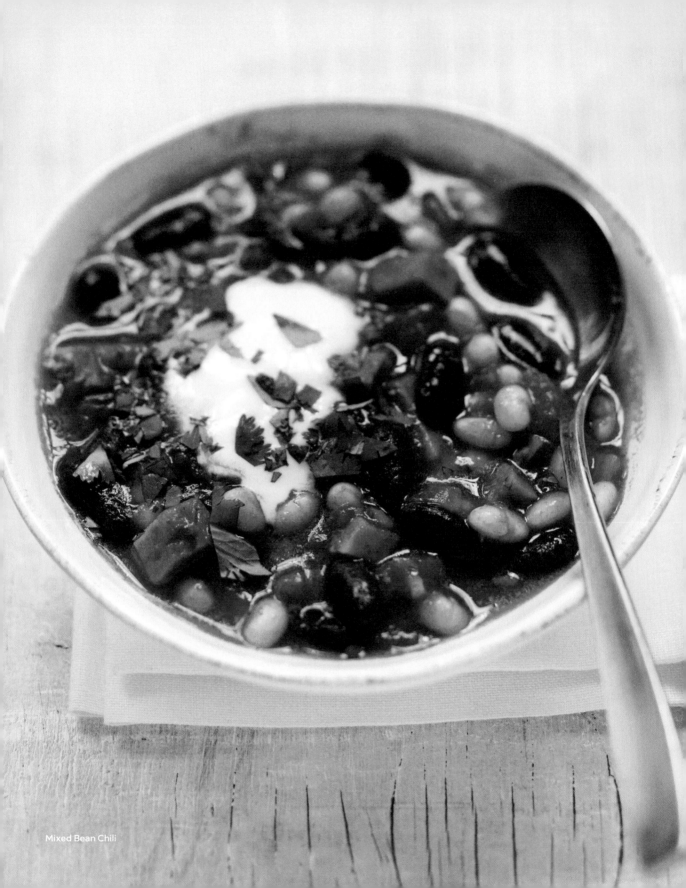

Mixed Bean Chili

CHAPTER EIGHT

Vegetarian and Vegan

VEGETARIAN EGG PIZZA

PREP TIME: 20 MINUTES · COOK TIME: 40 MINUTES
SERVES 4

You would be correct if you think this is a frittata with piles of vegetables, including plenty of healthy mushrooms. Especially low in calories, mushrooms are high in selenium, potassium, and vitamin D. Eating mushrooms along with foods with higher glycemic indexes can reduce the impact of sugar spikes and reduce cravings for sweet foods.

2 teaspoons olive oil, divided

1 zucchini, diced

1 red bell pepper, seeded and diced

1 yellow bell pepper, seeded and diced

1 red onion, diced

1 cup oyster mushrooms

½ cup sun-dried tomatoes

3 eggs

3 egg whites

1 tablespoon Dijon mustard

1 teaspoon chopped fresh thyme

½ cup arugula, divided

1. Preheat the oven to 375°F.

2. Line a baking sheet with parchment paper.

3. In a large bowl, toss together 1 teaspoon of oil, the zucchini, bell peppers, onion, mushrooms, and sun-dried tomatoes until well combined.

4. Spread the vegetables on the baking sheet and roast them for about 25 minutes, turning once, until they are tender and lightly caramelized.

5. Remove the vegetables from the oven and set aside.

6. In a small bowl, whisk together the eggs, egg whites, Dijon, and thyme.

7. Put a large skillet over medium heat, and add ½ teaspoon of oil.

8. Add half of the egg mixture to the skillet, and swirl the pan to spread the eggs evenly.

9. Cook for 5 to 7 minutes, until the eggs are just cooked through, and remove the skillet from the heat.

10. Top the eggs with half of the vegetable mixture, and sprinkle with half of the arugula.

11. Cut the pizza into 2 portions and keep warm.

12. Repeat, making another pizza with the remaining ingredients. Cut it into 2 portions, and serve.

SERVING TIP: Frittatas freeze beautifully, so divide up leftovers into desired serving sizes, and put the portions into sealed plastic containers. To reheat, microwave for a couple of minutes, and serve with a tossed salad.

PER SERVING Calories: 132; Carbs: 10g; Glycemic Load: 5; Fiber: 3g; Protein: 10g; Sodium: 205mg; Fat: 7g

RED LENTIL CURRY

PREP TIME: 20 MINUTES · COOK TIME: 50 MINUTES
SERVES 4

Lentils might seem like a forbidden food to those watching blood sugar levels, because these legumes are starchy in nature. However, lentils are very high in fiber, including insoluble fiber, which becomes gel-like when digested. This gel consistency slows the absorption of sugar, and leaves you feeling full and satisfied for long periods of time. Serve this curry over steamed brown rice.

1 tablespoon olive oil

1 sweet onion, chopped

2 teaspoons grated fresh ginger

1 teaspoon minced garlic

2 tablespoons red curry paste

½ teaspoon ground cumin

¼ teaspoon ground turmeric

Pinch cayenne

5 cups low-sodium vegetable broth

1½ cups red lentils, picked through and rinsed

¼ cup canned coconut milk

2 large tomatoes, diced

2 tablespoons chopped fresh cilantro, for garnish

1. Place a large saucepan over medium-high heat and add the olive oil.

2. Sauté the onion, ginger, and garlic for about 4 minutes, until softened and fragrant.

3. Add the curry paste, cumin, turmeric, and cayenne, and sauté for 1 minute.

4. Stir in the vegetable broth, lentils, and coconut milk, and bring the curry to a boil.

5. Reduce the heat to low and simmer the curry for about 45 minutes, until the lentils are tender and the liquid is mostly absorbed.

6. Add the tomatoes and stir to combine.

7. Serve the curry garnished with cilantro.

INGREDIENT TIP: If you have always used curry powder, you might be surprised by the strength of this spice blend in paste form. For a little extra kick, add more paste in very small increments, keeping in mind that the flavor will intensify as the dish cooks.

PER SERVING Calories: 407; Carbs: 58g; Glycemic Load: 14; Fiber: 25g; Protein: 22g; Sodium: 457mg; Fat: 10g

VEGGIE PECAN BURGERS

PREP TIME: 10 MINUTES, PLUS 30 MINUTES CHILLING TIME • COOK TIME: 15 MINUTES
SERVES 4

Vegetarian burgers, especially vegan products, have a bad reputation for being tasteless—or worse, containing strange textures or flavors. This burger is warmly spiced, with pecans adding a toasty sweetness. Pecans are high in healthy fat and fiber, and rank in the top 15 foods for antioxidant content, so enjoy these burgers as a regular meal choice. Substituting almonds or walnuts will yield impressive results, too.

2 teaspoons olive oil, divided

½ sweet onion, chopped

1 teaspoon minced garlic

1 cup canned chickpeas, rinsed
    and drained

1 cup chopped pecans

¼ cup fresh cilantro leaves, loosely packed

2 teaspoons low-sodium tamari sauce

½ teaspoon ground cumin

¼ teaspoon ground cinnamon

SERVING TIP: You can certainly serve these burgers traditionally, on a whole-grain bun, topped with sliced tomatoes, lettuce, and your favorite condiments. But if you prefer a lighter meal, these patties are just as good topped with a scoop of guacamole and accompanied by a salad.

1. Put a medium skillet over medium heat, and add 1 teaspoon of olive oil.

2. Sauté the onion and garlic for 5 to 6 minutes, until lightly caramelized.

3. Transfer the cooked vegetables to a food processor, and add the chickpeas, pecans, cilantro, tamari sauce, cumin, and cinnamon. Pulse the ingredients until the mixture is finely chopped and sticks together.

4. Divide the mixture into 4 equal burgers. Pat each burger so it measures about 3½ inches in diameter.

5. Put the burgers on a plate, covered, in the refrigerator for about 30 minutes to chill.

6. Preheat the oven to broil, and line a baking sheet with aluminum foil.

7. Brush both sides of the burgers with the remaining 1 teaspoon of olive oil, and put them on the baking sheet.

8. Broil the burgers for about 5 minutes per side, until the patties are golden and heated through, and serve.

PER SERVING Calories: 146; Carbs: 14g; Glycemic Load: 5; Fiber: 4g; Protein: 5g; Sodium: 206mg; Fat: 9g

MIXED BEAN CHILI

PREP TIME: 20 MINUTES • COOK TIME: 2½ HOURS

SERVES 6

Wintry days should end with a crackling fire and a steaming bowl of spicy, filling chili. This recipe is packed with nutritious legumes—high in fiber and protein, and low in calories. The fiber in legumes ensures the slow release of glucose into the blood, which prevents blood sugar spikes.

1 tablespoon olive oil

1 sweet onion, chopped

1 tablespoon minced garlic

¼ cup chili powder

1 teaspoon smoked sweet paprika

½ teaspoon ground cumin

2 cups canned navy beans, rinsed and drained

1 cup canned black beans, rinsed and drained

1 cup canned kidney beans, rinsed and drained

1 green bell pepper, seeded and diced

1 red bell pepper, seeded and diced

2 cups sodium-free vegetable broth

4 tomatoes, diced

1. Put a large stockpot over medium-high heat, and add the oil.

2. Sauté the onion and garlic for about 4 minutes, until softened.

3. Stir in the chili powder, paprika, and cumin, and stir to coat the vegetables.

4. Add the navy beans, black beans, kidney beans, peppers, stock, and tomatoes; stir to combine.

5. Bring the chili to a boil, reduce the heat to low, and simmer for 2 to 2½ hours, until the beans are very tender and the flavors mellow.

6. Remove from the heat, and serve.

SUBSTITUTION TIP: Chili can work with a combination of any types of beans, so don't feel constrained by the varieties listed here. Try adding black-eyed peas, lentils, or chickpeas to the pot.

PER SERVING Calories: 360; Carbs: 62g; Glycemic Load: 17; Fiber: 24g; Protein: 19g; Sodium: 325mg; Fat: 7g

VEGETABLE STEW

PREP TIME: 15 MINUTES • COOK TIME: 35 MINUTES
SERVES 4

What would a hearty stew be without chunks of bright carrot? This vegetable was once on the do-not-eat list for people with blood sugar issues because of its relatively high glycemic index. But many factors can affect this number, landing carrots anywhere on the scale between almost 70 for raw and 39 for cooked. Better to look at glycemic load instead, where carrots are in the much lower range of 3 for raw and 1 for cooked.

1 tablespoon olive oil

1 small sweet onion, peeled and chopped

2 celery stalks, chopped

2 teaspoons minced garlic

1 teaspoon ground cumin

½ teaspoon ground coriander

2 carrots, diced

1 red bell pepper, seeded and chopped

1 cup shredded green cabbage

2 cups sodium-free vegetable broth

½ cup pearl barley

2 large tomatoes, chopped

Pinch red pepper flakes

Pinch freshly ground black pepper

2 tablespoons chopped fresh parsley

7. Put a large stockpot over medium heat, and add the oil. Sauté the onion, celery, and garlic in the oil for about 4 minutes, until softened.

8. Add the cumin and coriander, and sauté for about 1 minute.

9. Add the carrots, red pepper, cabbage, vegetable broth, and barley.

10. Bring the stew to a boil, and then reduce the heat to low so it simmers.

11. Simmer for about 25 minutes, stirring often, until the barley and vegetables are tender.

12. Add the tomatoes, red pepper flakes, and freshly ground black pepper.

13. Simmer for 5 minutes, and serve sprinkled with parsley.

SUBSTITUTION TIP: Barley contains gluten, which can be a concern for anyone who has a sensitivity to this protein. The barley can be omitted entirely or replaced with brown rice to create a gluten-free dish.

PER SERVING Calories: 173; Carbs: 30g; Glycemic Load: 15; Fiber: 8g; Protein: 5g; Sodium: 57mg; Fat: 5g

STUFFED TOMATOES

PREP TIME: 30 MINUTES • COOK TIME: 40 MINUTES
SERVES 4

This is a tasty dish to bring to your next neighborhood or family gathering. The ingredients are inexpensive, and you can prepare it completely ahead of time—just warm it up when you arrive at your event. The red pepper in the filling not only adds color and sweetness but also vitamin A, vitamin C, and lycopene, which can reduce the risk of diabetes.

4 large, firm tomatoes

¼ teaspoon sea salt

1 teaspoon olive oil

½ sweet onion, chopped

1 teaspoon minced garlic

2 cups cannned green lentils, rinsed and drained

1 red bell pepper, seeded and chopped

1 cup shredded kale

1 teaspoon chopped fresh basil

1 teaspoon chopped fresh oregano

1 teaspoon lemon zest

½ cup sunflower seeds

Sea salt

Freshly ground black pepper

1. Cut the tops off the tomatoes and carefully scoop out the flesh, leaving empty shells. Use the tomato pulp for another recipe.

2. Lightly salt the insides of the tomatoes, and place them cut-side down on paper towels for about 30 minutes to purge extra juices.

3. While the tomatoes are purging, put a large skillet over medium-high heat, and add the olive oil.

4. Sauté the onion and garlic for about 3 minutes, until softened.

5. Stir in the lentils, red pepper, kale, basil, oregano, and lemon zest. Sauté the filling for 5 minutes, and stir in the sunflower seeds.

6. Season the filling with salt and freshly ground black pepper.

7. Preheat the oven to 350°F.

8. Place the tomatoes in an 8-by-8-inch baking dish, and spoon the filling into them evenly.

9. Bake the tomatoes for about 30 minutes, until they are softened and the filling is piping hot, and serve.

INGREDIENT TIP: Even if you purchase organic produce without pesticide residues, it is a good idea to scrub the lemon for this recipe well before zesting it. To protect them during shipping, lemons often have a wax coating you do not want to eat.

PER SERVING Calories: 271; Carbs: 42g; Glycemic Load: 16; Fiber: 19g; Protein: 16g; Sodium: 197mg; Fat: 5g

ZUCCHINI PASTA
with Savory Cherry Tomato Sauce

PREP TIME: 15 MINUTES • COOK TIME: 15 MINUTES

SERVES 4

There is nothing better than a dish that looks like it required hours of preparation when it actually took less than 30 minutes from start to finish. Here, the best technique is to have all your ingredients chopped, lined up, and ready to go, in the manner of professional chefs. For extra sweetness, add chopped roasted red bell pepper to the sauce.

1 teaspoon olive oil

2 teaspoons minced garlic

4 cups halved cherry tomatoes

½ cup chopped sun-dried tomatoes

½ cup chopped fresh basil

1 scallion, white and green parts, chopped

2 tablespoons chopped fresh oregano

Juice of 1 lemon

Pinch red pepper flakes

4 zucchini, julienned or cut into long
    noodles with a spiralizer

1. Put a large skillet over medium heat, and add the oil.

2. Sauté the garlic for 3 minutes.

3. Add the cherry tomatoes, sun-dried tomatoes, basil, scallion, oregano, lemon juice, and red pepper flakes to the skillet, and stir to combine.

4. Cook the sauce, stirring, for about 5 minutes, until the cherry tomatoes break up.

5. Add the zucchini to the skillet, and toss into the sauce with tongs for about 5 minutes, until the zucchini is tender. Serve.

COOKING TIP: If you enjoy dishes featuring noodle shapes, a spiralizer is a wonderful kitchen tool to consider purchasing. You can turn carrots, parsnips, zucchini, squash, and fruit into curling ribbons that are perfect to include in many dishes.

PER SERVING Calories: 89; Carbs: 17g; Glycemic Load: 9; Fiber: 6g; Protein: 5g; Sodium: mg; Fat: 2g

CAULIFLOWER-PECAN FRITTERS

PREP TIME: 25 MINUTES • COOK TIME: 16 MINUTES
SERVES 4

A fun recipe to prepare, these golden fritters are extremely enjoyable to eat. Cauliflower is an incredibly versatile ingredient that becomes soft and creamy when cooked, so it is often used as a substitute for mashed potatoes. On a nutritional level, cauliflower is an excellent source of vitamins C and K, fiber, and phytonutrients that can help you detox. Serve these fritters with a salad.

5 cups cauliflower florets, from about 1 medium head

1 cup grated carrot

2 eggs, beaten

¼ cup almond meal

¼ cup pumpkin seeds

¼ cup pecans, finely chopped

2 tablespoons chopped fresh parsley

1 tablespoon chopped fresh thyme

Juice of ½ lemon

⅛ teaspoon sea salt

⅛ teaspoon freshly ground black pepper

3 tablespoons olive oil

1. Put the cauliflower florets in a food processor, and pulse until the vegetable resembles rice. Transfer the cauliflower to a large bowl.

2. Stir in the carrot, eggs, almond meal, pumpkin seeds, pecans, parsley, thyme, lemon juice, salt, and pepper.

3. Mix until the mixture holds together when pressed. Form the mixture into 8 patties.

4. Put a large skillet over medium-high heat, and add the olive oil.

5. Cook the fritters in batches until they are golden brown on both sides, turning once, about 8 minutes total.

6. Serve 2 per person.

> **SERVING TIP:** If you like falafel, try these fritters stuffed into whole-grain pitas and topped with cool tzatziki and shredded lettuce. You can eat the fritters cold or warm, depending on your preference.

PER SERVING Calories: 271; Carbs: 13g; Glycemic Load: 3; Fiber: 6g; Protein: 9g; Sodium: 149mg; Fat: 22g

MOROCCAN-STYLE EGGPLANT

PREP TIME: 20 MINUTES, PLUS 30 MINUTES • COOK TIME: 25 MINUTES, PLUS 15 MINUTES
STANDING TIME

SERVES 4

North African cuisine is fragrant with warm spices and rich vegetable preparations. Eggplant is very popular because it's inexpensive and soaks up the other flavorings in the dish. Don't skip the first step, drawing out bitterness from the eggplant, or the dish will not taste as mellow. Coriander is beneficial when considering blood sugar; by helping stimulate the secretion of insulin, this spice can lower blood sugar levels.

2 eggplants (about 1½ pounds total)

⅛ teaspoon sea salt

2 tablespoons olive oil

½ sweet onion, chopped

3 teaspoons minced garlic

½ cup chopped fresh basil

1 pound tomatoes, chopped

½ cup sodium-free vegetable broth

½ teaspoon ground cumin

¼ teaspoon ground cinnamon

¼ teaspoon ground coriander

Pinch ground cloves

PER SERVING Calories: 162; Carbs: 23g; Glycemic Load: 14; Fiber: 12g; Protein: 4g; Sodium: 24mg; Fat: 8g

1. Cut the eggplant into 1-inch cubes, and toss in a bowl with the salt. Let the eggplant sit for 30 minutes to let the salt draw out the bitterness. Rinse the eggplant and pat it dry with a clean kitchen cloth.

2. Put a large skillet over medium-high heat, and add the olive oil.

3. Sauté the eggplant, onion, and garlic for 3 minutes, then cover the skillet and reduce the heat to low.

4. Sweat the eggplant for about 10 minutes, until soft.

5. Add the basil, tomatoes, broth, cumin, cinnamon, coriander, and cloves to the skillet, and stir to mix.

6. Sauté for about 10 minutes, until the sauce is thickened.

7. Let the dish stand for 15 minutes to mellow the flavors.

SERVING TIP: You can certainly eat this dish on its own like a stew, since it is filling and can stand alone in taste and texture. However, if you need to stretch the servings, spoon the braised eggplant over brown rice or cooked lentils.

ROASTED VEGETABLES
with Coconut Sauce

PREP TIME: 15 MINUTES • COOK TIME: 20 MINUTES
SERVES 4

Coconut milk is a smart choice for people who are insulin resistant or prediabetic. It has only 1 gram of carbohydrates per cup and is packed with healthy medium-chain saturated fatty acids, which can help fight disease and act as an anti-inflammatory. The high fat content can also slow the absorption of sugar.

2 carrots, cut into ½-inch chunks

1 head cauliflower, cut into florets

2 cups halved Brussels sprouts

2 cups green beans, cut into 1-inch pieces

1 red bell pepper, seeded and cut into 1-inch chunks

1 sweet onion, peeled and cut into eighths

1 tablespoon coconut oil

1 cup canned coconut milk

½ teaspoon ground turmeric

¼ teaspoon ground cardamom

Sea salt

2 tablespoons chopped fresh basil, for garnish

COOKING TIP: To save time, blanch the carrots in advance, and store them in plastic bags or containers in the refrigerator for up to 3 days.

1. Preheat the oven to 400°F.

2. Put a large saucepan filled with water over high heat, and bring to a boil.

3. Blanch the carrots for 5 minutes. Drain and transfer them to a large bowl.

4. Add the cauliflower, Brussels sprouts, green beans, red pepper, onion, and olive oil to the bowl. Toss to mix.

5. Transfer the vegetables to a baking sheet and spread them out.

6. Roast the vegetables, stirring at least once, for about 30 minutes, until they are lightly browned and tender.

7. While the vegetables are roasting, whisk together the coconut milk, turmeric, and cardamom. Season the sauce with salt and set aside.

8. When the vegetables are roasted, toss them in a large bowl with the coconut sauce, and serve sprinkled with basil.

PER SERVING Calories: 260; Carbs: 24g; Glycemic Load: 10; Fiber: 9g; Protein: 6g; Sodium: 126mg; Fat: 18g

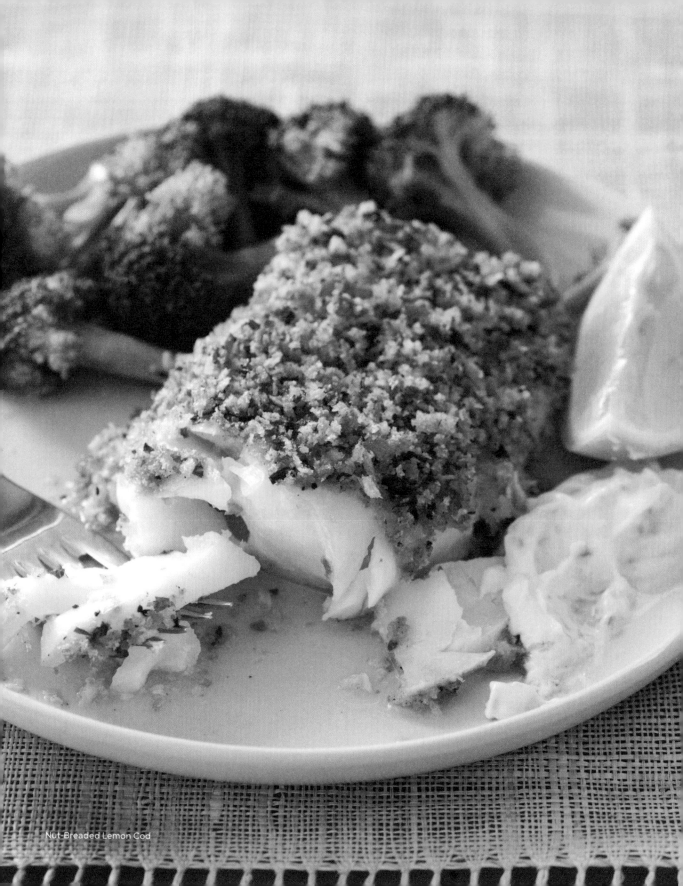

Nut-Breaded Lemon Cod

CHAPTER NINE

Fish and Seafood

GREEN CURRY MUSSELS

PREP TIME: 30 MINUTES • COOK TIME: 10 MINUTES
SERVES 2

Mussels probably seem like a restaurant meal, something you would order in a fine dining establishment because they are so tricky to make at home. But that couldn't be further from the truth—the only difficult step in preparing steamed mussels is cleaning them properly before cooking. Mussels are rich in vitamin B_{12}, protein, and manganese.

1 cup low-sodium vegetable broth

½ cup canned light coconut milk

1 (4-ounce) bottle clam juice

2 teaspoons green curry paste

Juice and zest of 1 lime

40 mussels (about 1 pound), scrubbed and debearded

¼ cup chopped fresh cilantro

Lime wedges, for garnish

1. In a large deep skillet over medium-high heat, stir together the vegetable broth, coconut milk, clam juice, curry paste, lime juice, and lime zest.

2. Bring the liquid to a boil, and add the mussels.

3. Cover and steam the mussels for about 5 minutes, until they open.

4. Discard any unopened mussels, and divide the remaining mussels between 2 bowls.

5. Pour the liquid left in the skillet into each bowl, and sprinkle the mussels with cilantro.

6. Garnish with lime wedges, and serve.

INGREDIENT TIP: Mussels are best purchased from September to April because they spawn in the spring, and the meat is not the best during that time. The cleaning process will be less extensive for cultivated mussels, because they are cultivated on hanging ropes, away from sand and grit.

PER SERVING Calories: 463; Carbs: 23g; Glycemic Load: 0; Fiber: 2g; Protein: 41g; Sodium: 876mg; Fat: 23g

TENDER CRAB CAKES

PREP TIME: 20 MINUTES, PLUS 1 HOUR CHILLING TIME · COOK TIME: 20 MINUTES
SERVES 4

These crab cakes are spectacular paired with Basil Salsa (page 75) or Wasabi Mayonnaise (page 74) for an extra kick of flavor. Crab is low in overall fat, and contains unsaturated heart-healthy fat along with chromium, which can improve blood sugar metabolism. Because it is lower on the food chain, with less contamination, crab usually presents a very low risk for mercury.

1 pound lump crabmeat, picked through carefully

½ cup almond flour

½ red bell pepper, minced

1 scallion, white and green parts, minced

¼ cup plain yogurt

1 tablespoon freshly squeezed lemon juice

1 teaspoon chopped fresh dill

Pinch red pepper flakes

3 tablespoons olive oil

1. In a large bowl, stir together the crab, almond flour, red pepper, scallion, yogurt, lemon juice, dill, and red pepper flakes until the mixture holds together when pressed. Add a little more almond flour if the mixture is too wet.

2. Form the crab mixture into 12 patties, and place them on a plate, covered, in the refrigerator for 1 hour.

3. Put a large skillet over medium heat, and add the olive oil.

4. Cook the crab cakes in batches for about 10 minutes total, turning the cakes once, until golden brown and heated completely through. Serve.

> **SUBSTITUTION TIP:** Crabmeat from your seafood counter is generally juicy and fresh; however, if this ingredient is unavailable, canned crab can be a good alternative. Just make sure you are using real crabmeat and not some strangely dyed imitation product.

PER SERVING Calories: 428; Carbs: 7g; Glycemic Load: 1; Fiber: 2g; Protein: 50g; Sodium: 662mg; Fat: 22g

JUICY SHRIMP
with Sweet and Spicy Dipping Sauce

PREP TIME: 15 MINUTES · COOK TIME: 10 MINUTES

SERVES 4

Grilled shrimp skewers are a most appealing summer dinner entrée, especially paired with a colorful salad such as Colorful Coleslaw (page 103) or a complex rice side dish. The Sriracha sauce in this recipe will elevate your mood—chile peppers boost endorphins and serotonin levels, creating a natural high. If you don't have a grill, you can broil the shrimp in the oven using the same timing.

½ pound sweet cherries, pitted

½ red bell pepper, chopped

1-inch piece ginger, peeled and grated

1 teaspoon Sriracha sauce

1 pound (16-20 count) shrimp, peeled and deveined, with tails left on

2 teaspoons olive oil

Sea salt

Freshly ground black pepper

1. In a blender, purée the sweet cherries, red pepper, ginger, and Sriracha sauce until smooth.

2. Store the sauce in the refrigerator in a sealed container until you wish to use it.

3. Preheat the grill to medium heat.

4. In a medium bowl, toss the shrimp and oil together, and lightly season the shrimp with salt and freshly ground black pepper.

5. Thread the shrimp onto 4 skewers and grill them, turning once, for about 10 minutes total, until the shrimp is opaque and cooked through.

6. Serve the shrimp with the dipping sauce.

PER SERVING Calories: 398; Carbs: 38g; Glycemic Load: 4; Fiber: 2g; Protein:41g; Sodium: 569mg; Fat: 8g

INGREDIENT TIP: Do not replace the Sriracha sauce with simple hot sauce or you will lose the complexity of flavor in this dish. Sriracha sauce is made from the same components as regular hot sauce, but it has a hint of sweetness as well, which pairs beautifully with the shrimp.

SHRIMP AND MUSSEL PAELLA

PREP TIME: 25 MINUTES • COOK TIME: 40 MINUTES

SERVES 6

Paella is a traditional Spanish dish featuring rice, saffron, meats, and seafood. This version does not have meat in it, but it certainly could pass for authentic. Paella is usually made in a special flat pan that can be found at most kitchen stores. But even without a special pan, this is a wonderfully satisfying one-pot meal that leaves time for your other pursuits.

1 tablespoon olive oil

1 sweet onion, chopped

2 teaspoons minced garlic

1 red bell pepper, seeded and chopped

1 cup brown rice

2 cups low-sodium chicken broth

1 cup chopped tomato

1 large pinch saffron threads, crushed

1 teaspoon chopped fresh thyme

¼ teaspoon freshly ground black pepper

⅛ teaspoon salt

1 pound (16-20 count) shrimp, peeled, deveined, and chopped

1 pound mussels, scrubbed and debearded ▸▸

1. Put a large skillet over medium heat and add the oil.

2. Sauté the onion and garlic for about 3 minutes, until softened.

3. Add the red pepper and sauté for 1 minute.

4. Stir in the rice, chicken broth, tomato, saffron, thyme, pepper, and salt.

5. Bring the mixture to a boil, then cover, reduce the heat, and simmer for about 30 minutes, until the rice is just tender.

6. Stir in the shrimp, and arrange the mussels on top of the rice.

7. Cover the skillet again, and cook for about 5 minutes, until the mussels have steamed open and the shrimp is cooked through.

8. Discard any unopened mussels, and serve immediately.

INGREDIENT TIP: Saffron is the dried stigma of the purple crocus flower. Real saffron is one of the most expensive spices in the world—it takes about 225,000 stigmas to produce 1 pound. So if you are purchasing saffron in your local grocery store for under $10 per gram, it is probably not saffron but dried parts of another flower.

PER SERVING Calories: 316; Carbs: 33g; Glycemic Load: 18; Fiber: 3g; Protein: 30g; Sodium: 479mg; Fat: 6g

SCALLOP AND VEGETABLE KEBABS

PREP TIME: 25 MINUTES · COOK TIME: 6 MINUTES
SERVES 4

Many home cooks assume scallops are difficult to prepare, most likely because an overcooked, rubbery scallop showed up on their plate in a restaurant. Scallops can easily be cooked too long, but if you watch the time carefully, you won't have a problem. Scallops are an excellent source of vitamin B_{12}, iodine, phosphorus, and protein.

1 tablespoon olive oil, plus more for brushing the grill

1 teaspoon chopped fresh thyme

1 teaspoon minced garlic

1 teaspoon lemon pepper

Pinch sea salt

1 pound sea scallops, rinsed and patted dry

1 large red bell pepper, seeded and cut into 8 pieces

1 large zucchini, cut into 8 chunks

1 large red onion, cut into 8 chunks

1 tablespoon chopped fresh parsley, for garnish

1. In a large bowl, stir together the olive oil, thyme, garlic, lemon pepper, and salt.

2. Add the scallops, red pepper, zucchini, and onion to the bowl, and toss to coat, taking care to keep the onion chunks from separating.

3. Thread the scallops and vegetables onto metal skewers, evenly dividing the ingredients.

4. Preheat a grill to medium heat, and brush the grates lightly with olive oil.

5. Grill the kebabs, turning once, for about 6 minutes total, until the scallops are lightly browned all over and cooked through.

6. Serve immediately.

SUBSTITUTION TIP: You can use bay scallops on your kebabs as well, but they are smaller than sea scallops and may not stay on the skewers as securely. Bay scallops have a slightly sweeter taste than their larger counterparts and are less expensive.

PER SERVING Calories: 161; Carbs: 10g; Glycemic Load: 3; Fiber: 2g; Protein: 20g; Sodium: 249mg; Fat: 5g

NUT-BREADED LEMON COD

PREP TIME: 15 MINUTES • COOK TIME: 10 MINUTES
SERVES 4

Simple food can often be dismissed as "boring," and one reason people fall off diets is because their palate is not used to tasting real food. This dish contains very few ingredients, but it is a lovely introduction to simple, healthy flavors. Appreciate the way the lemon enhances the cod. Really tasting your food can be an eye-opening experience that will help you stick to a healthy diet.

1 cup slivered almonds

1 teaspoon lemon zest

½ teaspoon chopped fresh thyme

Pinch sea salt

4 (6-ounce) cod fillets

2 eggs, beaten

Olive oil cooking spray

1. Preheat the oven to 450°F.

2. Line a baking sheet with aluminum foil.

3. Put the almonds, lemon zest, and thyme in a blender, and pulse until coarsely ground. Transfer the mixture to a plate, and stir in the salt.

4. Pat the fish dry with a paper towel.

5. Dredge a fish fillet in the beaten eggs, and press into the nut-lemon mixture to coat. Place the coated fish on the baking sheet.

6. Repeat with the other 3 fillets.

7. Lightly spray the breaded fish with olive oil.

8. Bake the fish for about 10 minutes, until it flakes easily when tested with a fork, and serve.

SUBSTITUTION TIP: Cod is a mild fish often found frozen in stores rather than fresh at the fish counter. Halibut, haddock, sole, and tilapia can all be used instead if you prefer to use a fresh fish.

PER SERVING Calories: 417; Carbs: 6g; Glycemic Load: 0; Fiber: 1g; Protein: 52g; Sodium: 274mg; Fat: 20g

POACHED HADDOCK with Herb Dressing

PREP TIME: 20 MINUTES · COOK TIME: 15 MINUTES

SERVES 4

Poached fish probably reminds you of brunch displays in fancy hotels where the poached salmon is dressed up in cucumber scales. This cooking method adds no fat, infuses the fish with herbs, and doesn't negatively affect the texture of the flesh. With no carbs at all, this dish has an impressive GL of zero.

FOR THE DRESSING

¼ cup olive oil

2 tablespoons freshly squeezed lemon juice

1 tablespoon lemon zest

1 tablespoon chopped fresh cilantro

2 teaspoons chopped fresh basil

1 teaspoon chopped fresh parsley

⅛ teaspoon salt

FOR THE FISH

6 cups water

1 lemon, cut into eighths

1 teaspoon chopped fresh thyme

½ teaspoon salt

½ teaspoon black peppercorns

4 (6-ounce) haddock fillets

TO MAKE THE DRESSING

In a small bowl, whisk together the olive oil, lemon juice, zest, cilantro, basil, parsley, and salt. Set aside.

TO MAKE THE FISH

1. In a large skillet, stir together the water, lemon wedges, thyme, salt, and peppercorns.

2. Bring the water to a boil, and then reduce the heat so the liquid simmers gently.

3. Add the haddock fillets, and cover the skillet.

4. Poach the fish for about 10 minutes, until it is just cooked through.

5. Remove the fish to a plate with a slotted spoon, and spoon the dressing over it. Serve.

> **COOKING TIP:** You can make this entire dish ahead of time, and serve the fish chilled for a leisurely brunch. The dressing is very nice on salads as well, so double the recipe and store some in the refrigerator for up to 1 week.

PER SERVING Calories: 299; Carbs: 0g; Glycemic Load: 0; Fiber: 0g; Protein: 41g; Sodium: 439mg; Fat: 14g

HALIBUT with Red Pepper Chutney

PREP TIME: 20 MINUTES • COOK TIME: 30 MINUTES
SERVES 4

Chutney has a wonderful old-fashioned ring to it, and it was originally created to use up produce to preserve for long winters. You can substitute peaches, nectarines, other bell peppers, and any type of herb to create chutney that suits your palate. Using toppings like this chutney opens the door to healthy protein dishes that both stick to your diet plan and require little fuss.

1 tablespoon olive oil, divided

1 teaspoon minced garlic

1 red bell pepper, seeded and chopped

1 cup chopped tomato

1 ripe plum, pitted and chopped

1 scallion, white and green parts, chopped

2 tablespoons apple cider vinegar

1 tablespoon chopped fresh thyme

4 (6-ounce) halibut fillets

Sea salt

Freshly ground black pepper

SUBSTITUTION TIP: The plum adds sweetness and a smooth texture to this chutney as it breaks down in the cooking process. If you can't find ripe plums, however, peaches, ripe nectarines, and pitted cherries would be equally scrumptious.

1. Put a small saucepan over medium heat, and add 1 teaspoon of olive oil.

2. Sauté the garlic and red pepper for 4 minutes.

3. Add the tomato, plum, scallion, apple cider vinegar, and thyme.

4. Stir to combine and bring the mixture to a simmer.

5. Reduce the heat to low and simmer the chutney for about 15 minutes, until the vegetables and fruit soften.

6. Pat the fish dry with paper towels, and lightly season both sides of the fillets with salt and freshly ground black pepper

7. Put a large skillet over medium-high heat, and add the remaining 2 teaspoons of oil.

8. Add the fillets and pan-sear for about 4 minutes per side, until the fish flakes easily when tested with a fork.

9. Serve the fish with the chutney.

PER SERVING Calories: 291; Carbs: 4g; Glycemic Load: 2; Fiber: 1g; Protein: 47g; Sodium: 182mg; Fat: 8g

OCEAN PERCH with Citrus-Fennel Slaw

PREP TIME: 25 MINUTES • COOK TIME: 6 MINUTES
SERVES 4

The citrus-spiked salad that accompanies this tender flaky fish just may become your new favorite starter or meal itself. The fresh taste and glorious presentation should perk up your senses, and its citrus components are packed with healthy vitamin C. Diabetic or prediabetic people's vitamin C levels are often low, so it is a good idea to keep your levels high.

1 orange

1 grapefruit

1 fennel bulb, shredded

2 celery stalks, shredded

1 tablespoon apple cider vinegar

½ teaspoon chopped fresh thyme

Sea salt

4 (6-ounce) ocean perch fillets

Freshly ground black pepper

1 tablespoon olive oil

INGREDIENT TIP: Perch is an often-overlooked fish, because it is not as well known as other species. It can originate from freshwater sources or from the Pacific Ocean, and is characterized by sweet, firm flesh. You can find it flash frozen if not available fresh.

1. Over a large bowl, cut the skin off the orange and grapefruit, leaving only the flesh. Section the fruit by cutting between the membranes. Squeeze the juice out of the membranes into the bowl.

2. Add the fennel, celery, apple cider vinegar, and thyme to the citrus. Season with salt, and toss to combine.

3. Pat the fish dry with paper towels, and season both sides lightly with salt and freshly ground black pepper.

4. Heat the olive oil in a large skillet over medium-high heat.

5. Add the fish to the skillet, and pan-sear, turning once, for about 3 minutes per side, until the fish flakes easily with a fork and is golden brown.

6. Serve the fish over a generous scoop of slaw.

PER SERVING Calories: 233; Carbs: 13g; Glycemic Load: 6; Fiber: 4g; Protein: 33g; Sodium: 252mg; Fat: 5g

PISTACHIO-CRUSTED SALMON

PREP TIME: 15 MINUTES • COOK TIME: 15 MINUTES
SERVES 4

Pistachios in their natural form are a light-green color—the bright red nuts you may find are dyed and definitely not suitable for a healthy diet. To cut costs, buy your pistachios in the shell, and shell them yourself for this recipe. Pistachios are high in protein, fiber, healthy monounsaturated fat, and vitamin E.

1 egg

2 tablespoons water

½ cup finely chopped unsalted dry-roasted pistachios

¼ cup ground almonds

½ teaspoon chopped fresh thyme

4 (6-ounce) salmon fillets

Sea salt

Freshly ground black pepper

1. Preheat the oven to 450°F.

2. In a small bowl, whisk together the egg and water.

3. In another small bowl, stir together the pistachios, ground almond, and thyme.

4. Pat the fish dry with paper towels. Season lightly with salt and freshly ground black pepper.

5. Dredge a fillet in the egg mixture, then in the nut mixture.

6. Transfer the fillet to a baking sheet, and repeat with the remaining fish.

7. Bake the fish for about 15 minutes, until it flakes easily when tested with a fork, and serve.

INGREDIENT TIP: Pacific-caught wild salmon from Alaska or British Columbia is the choice most highly recommended by health authorities. Atlantic salmon, by contrast, can be contaminated with mercury, and farm-raised fish are not as nutritious or tasty as their wild counterparts.

PER SERVING Calories: 368; Carbs: 6g; Glycemic Load: 0; Fiber: 3g; Protein: 39g; Sodium: 241mg; Fat: 22g

LEEK-BRAISED COD

PREP TIME: 15 MINUTES • COOK TIME: 15 MINUTES
SERVES 4

Fresh leeks that are 1 inch in diameter or less possess a sweet taste and become a superb shade of vibrant green when sautéed for a short time. You want to maintain that color because this dish is breathtaking when the leeks are combined with the sunny yellow broth. Sitting down to a fabulous healthy meal such as this at the end of a long day might be just what you need for emotional equilibrium.

2 tablespoons olive oil

2 leeks, white and light green parts, chopped and washed thoroughly

2 teaspoons minced garlic

2 cups low-sodium chicken broth

½ cup canned coconut milk

¼ teaspoon saffron threads, crushed

1 pound cod fillets, cut into 2-inch cubes

2 teaspoons chopped fresh thyme

1. In a large skillet, heat the oil over medium heat.

2. Sauté the leeks and garlic for about 5 minutes, until softened.

3. Stir in the broth, coconut milk, and saffron, and bring the sauce to a boil.

4. Add the fish, turning to coat, then reduce the heat to low and simmer, covered, for about 8 minutes, until the fish is tender.

5. Serve sprinkled with thyme.

SERVING TIP: You will be grateful for the quick execution of this dish, less than 30 minutes from start to finish. Try an equally speedy side dish of salad, quinoa, or simple steamed vegetables to round out the meal.

PER SERVING Calories: 253; Carbs: 9g; Glycemic Load: 2; Fiber: 2g; Protein: 22g; Sodium: 153mg; Fat: 15g

HERBED TROUT FILLETS

PREP TIME: 20 MINUTES • COOK TIME: 20 MINUTES
SERVES 4

Trout is very high in omega-3 fatty acids, protein, vitamin B_{12}, and vitamin B_6. This simple preparation beautifully complements the natural flavor of the fish with a bouquet of fresh herbs.

1 teaspoon olive oil

1 sweet onion, cut into eighths

4 (4-ounce) trout fillets

Sea salt

Freshly ground black pepper

1 tablespoon chopped fresh basil

1 teaspoon chopped fresh thyme

1 teaspoon chopped fresh oregano

1 teaspoon chopped fresh chives

¼ cup sodium-free vegetable broth

¼ cup freshly squeezed lemon juice

1. Preheat the oven to 350°F.

2. Lightly oil a 9-by-13-inch baking dish, and scatter the onion pieces in the bottom.

3. Pat the fish dry with paper towels, and lightly season with salt and freshly ground black pepper.

4. Lay the trout fillets on the onion, and sprinkle the basil, thyme, oregano, and chives over the fish.

5. Pour the broth and lemon juice over the fish, and cover the dish with aluminum foil.

6. Bake the fish for about 20 minutes, until it flakes easily with a fork.

7. Serve with the juices from the baking dish.

SUBSTITUTION TIP: For a creative alternative, try stuffing whole trout with herbs. Purchase whole, gutted trout, stuff the cavities with herb sprigs, then lay the fish on their side in the baking dish. Cook for about 10 minutes longer than this recipe recommends for fillets.

PER SERVING Calories: 243; Carbs: 4g; Glycemic Load: 1; Fiber: 1g; Protein: 31g; Sodium: 141mg; Fat: 11g

BROILED WILD SALMON
with Peach Salsa

PREP TIME: 30 MINUTES • COOK TIME: 15 MINUTES

SERVES 4

The sizzling fish and fresh salsa in this dish are so glorious to behold on the plate, you might have to force yourself to dig in. Cold-water fatty fish, such as wild-caught salmon, are one of the best sources of omega-3 fatty acids and protein. The combination helps slow the absorption of blood sugar as well as aids in protecting your cardiovascular system.

FOR THE SALSA

2 peaches, pitted and coarsely chopped

1 teaspoon grated fresh ginger

1 scallion, white and green parts, chopped

2 tablespoons chopped fresh cilantro

Juice and zest of 1 lime

Sea salt

FOR THE FISH

4 (6-ounce) wild salmon fillets

Sea salt

Freshly ground black pepper

1 tablespoon olive oil

TO MAKE THE SALSA

In a small bowl, stir together the peach, ginger, scallion, cilantro, lime juice, zest, and salt. Set aside.

TO MAKE THE FISH

1. Preheat the oven to broil.

2. Pat the salmon fillets dry with paper towels, and season both sides lightly with salt and freshly ground black pepper.

3. Place the salmon on a baking sheet, and drizzle the fish with olive oil.

4. Broil the salmon, turning once, for about 15 minutes total, until the fish flakes easily with a fork.

5. Serve with a generous spoonful of salsa.

COOKING TIP: Grilling is a good choice for wild salmon if you don't want to broil it, because the flesh of this fish is firm, so it stays together on the grill. The timing is the same for grilling, about 8 minutes per side on medium heat.

PER SERVING Calories: 341; Carbs: 5g; Glycemic Load: 3; Fiber: 1g; Protein: 36g; Sodium: 198mg; Fat: 19g

CURRY-MARINATED TILAPIA

PREP TIME: 10 MINUTES • COOK TIME: 30 MINUTES
SERVES 4

This is a variation on a familiar Indian chicken dish, tikka masala. The coconut oil coating in your baking dish will prevent sticking, while adding healthy fats, which are about 50 percent lauric acid. Coconut oil can help prevent heart disease, boost your energy, and support weight loss. Top the tilapia with sprigs of fresh cilantro for an elegant presentation.

1 teaspoon coconut oil

4 (4-ounce) tilapia fillets

1 cup canned coconut milk

½ cup plain yogurt

2 tablespoons red curry paste

½ teaspoon minced garlic

Pinch sea salt

1. Preheat the oven to 350°F.

2. Lightly grease a 9-by-13-inch baking dish with coconut oil.

3. Arrange the tilapia fillets in the baking dish in a single layer.

4. In a medium bowl, whisk together the coconut milk, yogurt, curry paste, garlic, and salt.

5. Spread the yogurt mixture over the fish, and bake for about 30 minutes, until the fish is just cooked through. Serve.

INGREDIENT TIP: Coconut milk comes in many different forms, from thick canned products to a thinner drink found in cartons in the milk section of the grocery store. You want the canned version for this recipe because it is similar to heavy cream, especially when combined with tangy yogurt.

PER SERVING Calories: 293; Carbs: 7g; Glycemic Load: 1; Fiber: 1g; Protein: 24g; Sodium: 519mg; Fat: 19g

SALMON BURGERS

PREP TIME: 15 MINUTES, PLUS 30 MINUTES CHILLING TIME • COOK TIME: 12 MINUTES
SERVES 4

Fish burgers and fingers were all the rage in the 1980s because they were inexpensive and quick, which means they have horrible connotations for many adults today. But these fresh salmon burgers bear no resemblance to the notorious fish burgers of the eighties, so you can banish all those bad memories. These burgers are free of all the undesirable additives and high sodium, so they support a healthy diet.

1 pound salmon fillets, finely chopped

½ cup ground almonds

1 scallion, white and green parts, finely chopped

1 egg, beaten

½ red bell pepper, minced

½ teaspoon minced garlic

½ teaspoon grated fresh ginger

Pinch sea salt

Pinch freshly ground black pepper

2 tablespoons olive oil

1. In a large bowl, mix together the salmon, ground almonds, scallion, egg, red pepper, garlic, ginger, salt, and pepper, until it holds together when squeezed.

2. Form the mixture into 4 patties about ½ inch thick, and place the patties on a plate in the refrigerator for about 30 minutes to firm up.

3. Put a large skillet over medium heat, and add the olive oil.

4. Cook the salmon patties for about 6 minutes per side, turning once, until they are golden brown all over and cooked through. Serve.

SUBSTITUTION TIP: Fresh ginger has a lovely bite to it, with no bitterness or real heat. If possible, do not substitute dried ground ginger in this recipe, because the taste will not be the same; however, if dried is all you have available, use ¼ teaspoon.

PER SERVING Calories: 302; Carbs: 4g; Glycemic Load: 1; Fiber: 2g; Protein: 26g; Sodium: 175mg; Fat: 21g

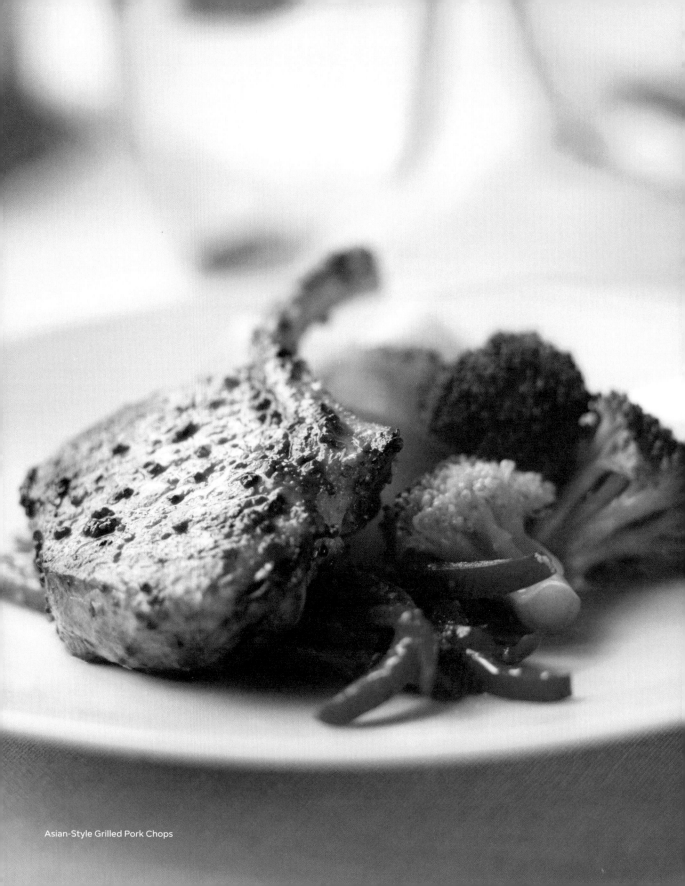

Asian-Style Grilled Pork Chops

Poultry and Meat

GINGER RICE NOODLES
with Chicken

PREP TIME: 20 MINUTES, PLUS 1 HOUR SOAKING TIME • COOK TIME: 15 MINUTES
SERVES 4

The only thing missing when you sit down to these noodles will be the take-out container. The base flavors of this dish are ginger and garlic, powerhouses of flavor and healthy benefits. Both these fragrant ingredients can improve insulin sensitivity as well as lower cholesterol and blood pressure. Crush or chop these ingredients 10 minutes before using to release the active compounds, or you may lose the health-boosting properties.

4 ounces dried rice noodles

2 teaspoons olive oil

1 scallion, white and green parts, finely chopped

2 teaspoons grated fresh ginger

2 teaspoons minced garlic

2 cups canned coconut milk

1 cup low-sodium chicken broth

Juice and zest of 1 lime

2 tablespoons chopped fresh cilantro

2 carrots, shredded

2 cups snow peas, julienned

2 (5-ounce) cooked boneless, skinless chicken breast halves, cut into bite-size pieces

3 tablespoons chopped peanuts

1. Put the rice noodles in a large bowl, and cover with water by about 2 inches. Let the noodles soak for about 1 hour, until softened.

2. Put a large skillet over medium heat, and add the oil.

3. Sauté the scallion, ginger, and garlic for about 3 minutes, until softened.

4. Stir in the coconut milk, chicken broth, lime juice, lime zest, and cilantro.

5. Bring the sauce to a boil, and add the carrots, snow peas, rice noodles, and chicken. Simmer the vegetables and chicken for about 7 minutes, until heated through and tender.

6. Serve sprinkled with chopped peanuts.

> **SUBSTITUTION TIP:** Top this dish with roasted pumpkin seeds instead, if you have a peanut allergy or are serving it to a guest with this dietary concern. Toasting the seeds will add rich flavor and a delightful crunch.

PER SERVING Calories: 554; Carbs: 25g; Glycemic Load: 19; Fiber: 7g; Protein: 29g; Sodium: 145mg; Fat: 35g

10

CHICKEN VEGETABLE MEATLOAF

PREP TIME: 15 MINUTES • COOK TIME: 50 MINUTES

SERVES 4

Butternut squash is on the eat-in-moderation list for insulin resistance, because it is a starchy vegetable and sweet. However, this colorful vegetable is high in vitamin E, a fat-soluble antioxidant that improves insulin action, so you'll reduce your insulin resistance naturally by eating foods high in this nutrient.

1 pound lean ground chicken

½ cup almond flour

1 egg, beaten

1 cup finely grated butternut squash

1 red bell pepper, seeded and finely chopped

1 scallion, white and green parts, finely chopped

1 teaspoon grated fresh ginger

1 teaspoon minced garlic

Pinch sea salt

Pinch freshly ground black pepper

1. Preheat the oven to 350°F.

2. Line an 8-by-4-inch loaf pan with parchment paper.

3. In a large bowl, mix all the ingredients together until well combined.

4. Pack the meatloaf into the loaf pan, and bake for about 50 minutes, until the meatloaf is cooked through and golden on top.

5. Remove the meatloaf from the oven and let it stand for 10 minutes.

6. Drain off any excess grease, and serve.

SUBSTITUTION TIP: Ground turkey, pork, beef, and veal, or a combination of these, will all work in this recipe instead of ground chicken. If you use beef or veal, omit the ginger, and replace it with ¼ cup finely chopped onion.

PER SERVING Calories: 205; Carbs: 5g; Glycemic Load: 6; Fiber: 2g; Protein: 26g; Sodium: 213mg; Fat: 9g

ARTICHOKE-CHICKEN BAKE

PREP TIME: 15 MINUTES • COOK TIME: 40 MINUTES
SERVES 4

There is something appealing—not to mention convenient—about a dinner prepared in a single, large dish. The flavors meld together, and you get a little bit of everything in each delicious bite. This recipe has lots of kale, which is rich in magnesium, like most dark leafy greens, and can positively affect the body's insulin receptors, improving glucose tolerance and insulin sensitivity.

2 teaspoons olive oil, divided

4 (5-ounce) boneless, skinless chicken breast halves

Sea salt

Freshly ground black pepper

½ sweet onion, chopped

1 teaspoon minced garlic

6 cups shredded kale

1 cup chopped artichoke hearts

½ cup canned coconut milk

½ cup plain yogurt

1 teaspoon ground coriander

¼ teaspoon ground cardamom

INGREDIENT TIP: Look for marinated artichoke hearts in jars, because the canned products can be soggy and have a sharp flavor.

1. Preheat the oven to 375°F.

2. Lightly grease an 8-by-8-inch baking dish with 1 teaspoon of olive oil, and arrange the chicken breasts in a single layer.

3. Lightly season the breasts with salt and pepper, and bake them for about 15 minutes, until they are almost cooked through.

4. While the chicken is baking, put a large skillet over medium heat, and add the remaining 1 teaspoon of olive oil.

5. Sauté the onion and garlic for about 3 minutes, until tender.

6. Add the kale and sauté for about 5 minutes, until wilted.

7. Remove the skillet from the heat, and stir in the artichoke hearts, coconut milk, yogurt, coriander, and cardamom, until well mixed.

8. Spoon the mixture over the baked chicken, and put the dish back in the oven for 20 to 25 minutes, until the top is lightly browned and the sauce is bubbly. Serve.

PER SERVING Calories: 456; Carbs: 20g; Glycemic Load: 5; Fiber: 5g; Protein: 48g; Sodium: 289mg; Fat: 20g

BREADED CHICKEN with Mustard

PREP TIME: 20 MINUTES • COOK TIME: 10 MINUTES
SERVES 4

The sauce for this chicken is rich and savory, but you can easily serve the chicken cutlets without it, or with a scoop of fresh salsa for a lighter dish. The chicken can be made ahead of time and eaten cold as well, so this provides a convenient meal on days when you're rushing out the door.

¼ cup almond flour

1 teaspoon lemon zest

⅛ teaspoon freshly ground black pepper

4 (4-ounce) boneless, skinless chicken breast halves

2 tablespoons olive oil

1 scallion, white and green parts, chopped

2 tablespoons grainy mustard

2 teaspoons chopped fresh tarragon

Juice of 1 lemon

Sea salt

SUBSTITUTION TIP: Grainy mustard or Pommery mustard has plump mustard seeds and a gorgeous complex flavor that cannot be replaced by plain yellow mustard. The only substitution that will work in this recipe is real Dijon mustard.

1. In a shallow dish, stir together the almond flour, lemon zest, and pepper. Set aside.

2. Put the chicken breasts between two pieces of plastic wrap, and pound them about ¼ inch thick.

3. Dredge the chicken breasts in the almond mixture, coating both sides.

4. Put a large skillet on medium heat, and add the oil.

5. Pan-sear the chicken in batches for about 4 minutes per side, until cooked through and golden brown on both sides.

6. Remove the chicken to a plate, and cover it loosely with foil to keep warm.

7. Add the scallions to the skillet, and sauté for 1 minute.

8. Add the mustard, tarragon, and lemon juice, and stir to combine.

9. Season the sauce with salt, and serve over the chicken.

PER SERVING Calories: 293; Carbs: 1g; Glycemic Load: 0; Fiber: 0g; Protein: 33g; Sodium: 191mg; Fat: 17g

GOLDEN CHICKEN
with Spicy Refried Beans

PREP TIME: 20 MINUTES • COOK TIME: 35 MINUTES

SERVES 4

Minerals and vitamins are extremely important when you're trying to manage insulin resistance. Your first line of defense is to consume these crucial nutrients by eating the right foods, such as legumes like pinto beans. Pinto beans are high in potassium, which can improve insulin sensitivity and the effectiveness of the insulin in the body.

1 tablespoon olive oil, divided

1 sweet onion, chopped

1 teaspoon minced garlic

1 jalapeño pepper, finely chopped

1 (15-ounce) can pinto beans, rinsed and drained

1 tomato, chopped

1 teaspoon chili powder

Juice of 1 lime

2 teaspoons ground cumin

2 teaspoons ground coriander

Pinch cayenne

Pinch sea salt

Pinch freshly ground black pepper

1 pound boneless, skinless chicken breasts, cut into 1-inch strips lengthwise

1. Put a large saucepan over medium heat, and add 1 teaspoon of oil.

2. Sauté the onion and garlic for about 3 minutes, until softened.

3. Add the jalapeño, pinto beans, tomato, chili powder, and lime juice to the saucepan, stirring to mix.

4. Cook, stirring frequently, for about 20 minutes, until the beans are very tender.

5. Remove the saucepan from the heat, and using a potato masher, mash the bean mixture until creamy. Set aside.

6. In a medium bowl, stir together the cumin, coriander, cayenne, salt, and freshly ground black pepper until blended. Add the chicken strips, and toss to coat with the spices.

7. Put a large skillet over medium-high heat, and heat the remaining 2 teaspoons of olive oil.

8. Pan-sear the chicken for about 10 minutes, until it is completely cooked through and golden brown on all sides.

9. Serve the chicken strips on the refried beans.

SERVING TIP: This is a complete, filling meal with side dish and chicken all in one. To further enhance the dish's presentation and flavor, try adding fresh shredded lettuce, chopped tomato, and a splash of hot sauce.

PER SERVING Calories: 420; Carbs: 32g; Glycemic Load: 6; Fiber: 11g; Protein: 43g; Sodium: 168mg; Fat: 13g

TURKEY AND BEAN CHILI

PREP TIME: 15 MINUTES • COOK TIME: 55 MINUTES
SERVES 4

Chili would be nothing without a hefty scoop of chili powder, so feel free to experiment with the quantity of this spice to produce the perfect balance of heat and flavor. Chili powder is beneficial for insulin resistance because it is high in manganese—especially desirable, since low levels of manganese can impair glucose metabolism and weaken the effectiveness of insulin.

1 teaspoon olive oil

1 pound lean ground turkey breast

1 sweet onion, chopped

1 jalapeño pepper, finely chopped

2 teaspoons minced garlic

¼ cup chili powder

2 teaspoons ground cumin

Pinch cayenne powder

4 tomatoes, chopped

1 cup canned red kidney beans, rinsed and drained

1 cup canned black beans, rinsed and drained

1 cup canned chickpeas, rinsed and drained

1. Put a large stockpot over medium heat and add the oil.

2. Sauté the turkey for about 6 minutes, until cooked through.

3. Add the onion, jalapeño pepper, and garlic, and sauté for about 4 minutes, until tender.

4. Stir in the chili powder, cumin, cayenne, tomatoes, red kidney beans, black beans, and chickpeas.

5. Bring the chili to a boil, then reduce the heat to low and simmer for about 45 minutes, until the flavors mellow. Serve.

INGREDIENT TIP: Cumin can be purchased in ground form at any supermarket, but toasting whole cumin seeds and grinding your own produces a spectacular flavor. Put the seeds in a small saucepan over medium heat, and swirl them for about 20 minutes, until very fragrant and lightly golden, then grind and use.

PER SERVING Calories: 377; Carbs: 41g; Glycemic Load: 15; Fiber: 14g; Protein: 43g; Sodium: 298mg; Fat: 7g

10

BRAISED PORK CUTLETS with Spinach

PREP TIME: 20 MINUTES • COOK TIME: 25 MINUTES

SERVES 4

Schnitzel, another name for these crispy golden cutlets, is a traditional dish often served with apples and braised vegetables. Here, the cutlets are braised along with the vegetables to create a main course and side dish all in one skillet. Lean meats like pork are a good source of chromium, an important mineral for the proper metabolism of carbohydrates and the effective functioning of insulin in the body.

4 (4-ounce) boneless pork chops, pounded to ½-inch thickness

Sea salt

Freshly ground black pepper

¼ cup almond flour

2 tablespoons olive oil

2 teaspoons minced garlic

1 cup low-sodium chicken broth

2 tomatoes, diced

8 cups baby spinach

1. Lightly season the cutlets with sea salt and freshly ground black pepper.

2. In a shallow dish, dredge the cutlets in the almond flour.

3. Put a large, deep skillet over medium heat, and add the olive oil.

4. Brown the pork chops on both sides, turning once, for about 6 minutes.

5. Remove the cutlets from the skillet, and add the garlic.

6. Sauté for 1 minute, then stir in the broth, tomatoes, and spinach.

7. Bring the liquid to a boil, tossing the spinach with tongs until it is wilted.

8. Reduce the heat to medium-low and return the cutlets to the skillet. Cover and simmer for about 15 minutes, until tender. Serve.

SUBSTITUTION TIP: If you have tree nut allergies, replace the almond flour with rice flour or quinoa flour. These substitutions will not brown as much, and the flavor will be slightly different. You can also pan-sear the pork with just salt and pepper.

PER SERVING Calories: 263; Carbs: 6g; Glycemic Load: 2; Fiber: 2g; Protein: 33g; Sodium: 192mg; Fat: 12g

10

MEDITERRANEAN PORK CHOPS

PREP TIME: 10 MINUTES, PLUS 30 MINUTES MARINATING TIME • COOK TIME: 35 MINUTES
SERVES 4

Pork is often referred to as the "other white meat" for its color when cooked, and because it falls between chicken and beef on a nutritional scale. Pork is high in protein, low in fat, and a good source of vitamin D, which can help boost insulin sensitivity and reduce belly fat.

4 (4-ounce) pork loin chops

Sea salt

Freshly ground black pepper

1 tablespoon minced garlic

1 teaspoon chopped fresh rosemary

1 teaspoon chopped fresh oregano

1. Season the pork chops lightly on both sides with salt and freshly ground black pepper.

2. In a small bowl, stir together the garlic, rosemary, and oregano.

3. Rub the pork chops all over with the garlic paste, and let them stand for 30 minutes at room temperature.

4. Preheat the oven to 350°F.

5. Place the pork chops on a baking sheet, and roast them, turning once, for about 35 minutes. Serve.

SERVING TIP: Simple flavorings and juicy pork create an elegant, satisfying dish that combines well with richer side dishes. Try pairing these chops with Beans with Sun-Dried Tomatoes (page 124) and Lemon Asparagus (page 126) for a gorgeous, balanced plate.

PER SERVING Calories: 368; Carbs: 1g; Glycemic Load: 0; Fiber: 0g; Protein: 26g; Sodium: 138mg; Fat: 28g

ASIAN-STYLE GRILLED PORK CHOPS

PREP TIME: 10 MINUTES, PLUS 1 HOUR MARINATING TIME • COOK TIME: 12 MINUTES
SERVES 4

Pork tastes spectacular when caramelized lightly with a sweet marinade or glaze. Don't shake off the excess marinade from the chops in this recipe: You want it to form a flavorsome sauce while on the grill. The chops can just as easily be broiled or roasted in the oven. Pork is low in fat while high in protein, thiamine, niacin, and phosphorus.

2 tablespoons sesame oil

2 tablespoons low-sodium tamari sauce

1 teaspoon minced garlic

1 teaspoon grated fresh ginger

1 teaspoon honey

1 teaspoon chili sauce

4 (5-ounce) center-cut pork chops, trimmed of fat

1. In a medium bowl, whisk together the sesame oil, tamari sauce, garlic, ginger, honey, and chili sauce.

2. Add the pork chops to the marinade, and turn to coat. Cover the bowl and marinate for 1 hour.

3. Preheat the grill to medium-high.

4. Grill the pork chops for about 6 minutes per side, turning once, until they are just cooked through. Serve.

INGREDIENT TIP: Made from the by-products of miso paste, tamari sauce is a Japanese version of soy sauce that provides a gluten-free option for many people. It contains less sodium than soy sauce and has an interesting, slightly sweet flavor.

PER SERVING Calories: 243; Carbs: 3g; Glycemic Load: 2; Fiber: 0g; Protein: 31g; Sodium: 345mg; Fat: 12g

10

PAN-SEARED LAMB CHOPS
with Sun-Dried Tomato Tapenade

PREP TIME: 30 MINUTES • COOK TIME: 25 MINUTES, PLUS 10 MINUTES RESTING TIME
SERVES 4

Shiny, black Kalamata olives are often cured in salt rather than soaked in brine, so they are mellow in flavor and less salty. Look closely at the label, because real Kalamata olives come from a particular region in Greece. Olives contain an impressively high quantity of phytonutrients, so these unassuming little fruits can have a positive impact on almost every system in the body.

FOR THE TAPENADE

½ cup sun-dried tomatoes

¼ cup pitted Kalamata olives

2 teaspoons minced garlic

2 tablespoons chopped fresh basil

1 tablespoon freshly squeezed lemon juice

1 tablespoon olive oil

FOR THE LAMB CHOPS

2 (1-pound) racks French-cut lamb chops (6 bones each)

Sea salt

Freshly ground black pepper

1 tablespoon olive oil

TO MAKE THE TAPENADE

1. In a blender, mix the sun-dried tomatoes, olives, garlic, basil, lemon juice, and olive oil, and pulse until the mixture is puréed but still slightly chunky.

2. Transfer the tapenade to a sealed container, and store in the refrigerator until needed. It can keep for up to 1 week.

TO MAKE THE LAMB CHOPS

1. Bring the tapenade to room temperature.

2. Preheat the oven to 450°F.

3. Season the lamb racks on both sides with salt and freshly ground black pepper.

4. Put a large ovenproof skillet over medium-high heat, and add the olive oil.

5. Pan-sear the racks on both sides and the bottoms for about 5 minutes total.

6. Arrange the racks in the skillet, bone-side down, and roast in the oven for about 20 minutes for medium-rare (internal temperature 125°F).

7. Let the lamb rest for 10 minutes, and then cut the racks into chops. Arrange 3 chops per plate, and spoon the tapenade over them.

INGREDIENT TIP: French-cut lamb racks have the flesh scraped out from between the upper bones so that they are bare, making an attractive presentation. This technique can be difficult to manage on your own, so ask your butcher to take care of this preparation step for you.

PER SERVING Calories: 471; Carbs: 5g; Glycemic Load: 4; Fiber: 1g; Protein: 46g; Sodium: 434mg; Fat: 26g

GREEK-STYLE LAMB ROAST

PREP TIME: 20 MINUTES • COOK TIME: 50 MINUTES, PLUS 15 MINUTES RESTING TIME
SERVES 8

In North America, where beef reigns supreme, lamb is not a protein often seen in home kitchens. Lamb tends to be more popular in countries that do not have the land or the water to support cattle. Yet lamb is not only delicious but very high in protein, which is digested more slowly than carbs and has no impact on blood sugar.

1 large onion, peeled and sliced

1 lamb leg roast, about 2 pounds

Sea salt

Freshly ground black pepper

1 tablespoon olive oil

1 tablespoon chopped fresh oregano

Juice and zest of 1 lemon

2 teaspoons minced garlic

1. Preheat the oven to 350°F.

2. Layer the onion slices in a large roasting pan.

3. Lightly season the lamb all over with salt and freshly ground black pepper, and place it on the onion slices.

4. In a small bowl, whisk together the olive oil, oregano, lemon juice, lemon zest, and garlic until blended.

5. Brush the lamb generously with the lemon mixture.

6. Roast for 50 minutes for medium (internal temperature 135°F to 140°F).

7. Let the lamb rest for 15 minutes, then slice and serve.

SERVING TIP: A traditional side dish for lamb is often roast potatoes, which are not appropriate for the Insulin Resistance Diet. Try Roasted Brussels Sprouts with Walnuts (page 125) instead, along with fluffy steamed brown rice.

PER SERVING Calories: 326; Carbs: 2g; Glycemic Load: 0; Fiber: 1g; Protein: 19g; Sodium: 97mg; Fat: 27g

10

MARINATED VENISON STEAKS

PREP TIME: 10 MINUTES, PLUS 2 HOURS MARINATING TIME • COOK TIME: 12 MINUTES
SERVES 4

Cherries might seem like an unlikely ingredient in a venison marinade, but this rich meat pairs very well with fruit. Cherries contain anthocyanins, which can boost insulin production by as much as 50 percent. Anthocyanins are also powerful antioxidants, so they can protect the body from inflammation, another trigger for insulin resistance.

¼ cup olive oil

¼ cup apple cider vinegar

¼ cup pitted cherries

2 tablespoons low-sodium tamari sauce

2 tablespoons freshly squeezed
   lemon juice

1 tablespoon grainy mustard

1 tablespoon chopped fresh parsley

1 teaspoon minced garlic

4 (5-ounce) venison tenderloin steaks

COOKING TIP: Do not marinate the venison for longer than 2 hours, because the acid in the marinade can tighten up the muscle fibers in the meat, making it tough. Venison should not be cooked to more than medium doneness; this very lean meat can become dry if cooked well done.

1. Combine the olive oil, apple cider vinegar, cherries, tamari sauce, lemon juice, grainy mustard, parsley, and garlic in a blender, and pulse to blend.

2. Transfer the marinade to a sealable plastic bag.

3. Add the venison to the bag, press out all the air, and seal.

4. Marinate the venison in the refrigerator, turning the bag several times, for 2 hours.

5. Preheat the grill to medium-high.

6. Remove the tenderloin from the refrigerator, and discard the marinade.

7. Grill the venison for about 6 minutes per side for medium-rare (internal temperature about 145°F).

8. Let the venison rest for 10 minutes, and serve.

PER SERVING Calories: 278; Carbs: 2g; Glycemic Load: 0; Fiber: 0g; Protein: 32g; Sodium: 335mg; Fat: 14g

MARINARA-BRAISED MEATBALLS

PREP TIME: 25 MINUTES • COOK TIME: 1 HOUR
SERVES 8

Your kitchen will smell like an Italian restaurant's while this sauce and the meatballs simmer on the stove. These meatballs are packed with protein and vitamin B_{12}, as well as about 37 milligrams of zinc per pound of ground beef. It's important to keep your zinc level high when managing insulin resistance; a deficiency in this mineral can contribute to reduced insulin sensitivity. Serve the meatballs and sauce over zucchini "noodles" made with a spiralizer.

FOR THE SAUCE

2 tablespoons olive oil

1 sweet onion, chopped

1 tablespoon minced garlic

8 large tomatoes, peeled and cut into large chunks

1 cup low-sodium chicken broth

2 tablespoons balsamic vinegar

1 tablespoon chopped fresh basil

1 tablespoon chopped fresh oregano

1 bay leaf

¼ teaspoon sea salt

¼ teaspoon freshly ground black pepper

¼ teaspoon red pepper flakes

FOR THE MEATBALLS

1 pound lean ground beef

1 pound lean ground pork

1 cup almond flour

1 egg

1 teaspoon minced garlic

1 teaspoon chopped fresh oregano

1 teaspoon chopped fresh parsley

¼ teaspoon sea salt

¼ teaspoon freshly ground black pepper

TO MAKE THE SAUCE

1. Put a large stockpot over medium heat, and add the olive oil.

2. Sauté the onion and garlic for about 3 minutes, until softened.

3. Stir in the tomatoes, chicken broth, balsamic vinegar, basil, oregano, bay leaf, salt, pepper, and red pepper flakes.

4. Bring the sauce to a boil, reduce the heat to low, and simmer for 30 minutes to mellow the flavors.

TO MAKE THE MEATBALLS

1. While the sauce is simmering, in a large bowl, combine the beef, pork, almond flour, egg, garlic, oregano, parsley, salt, and pepper until very well mixed.

2. Roll the mixture into meatballs about 1 inch in diameter.

3. Drop the raw meatballs into the sauce one by one, and continue simmering for about 30 minutes, stirring occasionally, until the meatballs are cooked through.

4. Remove the bay leaf, and serve.

COOKING TIP: This sauce and meatballs can be made in advance and frozen for up to 1 month in a sealed container. Cooking the meatballs in the sauce infuses the tomatoes with a rich beef taste and creates a truly authentic Italian culinary experience.

PER SERVING Calories: 284; Carbs: 10g; Glycemic Load: 4; Fiber: 3g; Protein: 32g; Sodium: 211mg; Fat: 13g

10

HEARTY BEEF AND NAVY BEAN STEW

PREP TIME: 20 MINUTES • COOK TIME: 1 HOUR, 15 MINUTES

SERVES 4

Navy beans are a buttery-textured legume that was a staple in the US Navy at the beginning of the twentieth century. Because of their high fiber and protein content, legumes are a healthy choice when attempting to increase insulin sensitivity. Try to include legumes regularly in your diet to improve your cholesterol and insulin levels.

1 tablespoon olive oil

1 (10-ounce) boneless round steak, cut into ½-inch cubes

2 cups quartered mushrooms

1 sweet onion, chopped

2 teaspoons minced garlic

2 tomatoes, chopped

2 carrots, diced

1 sweet potato, diced

1 cup sodium-free beef broth

2 bay leaves

1 tablespoon chopped fresh thyme

1 cup canned navy beans, rinsed and drained

2 cups green beans, cut into 1-inch pieces

Sea salt

Freshly ground black pepper

1. Put a large stockpot over medium heat, and add the oil.

2. Brown the beef in batches, and remove the browned beef to a plate with a slotted spoon.

3. Add the mushrooms, onion, and garlic, and sauté for about 5 minutes, until the vegetables are softened.

4. Stir in the reserved meat with the juices from the plate, and the tomatoes, carrots, sweet potato, beef broth, bay leaves, and thyme.

5. Bring the liquid to a boil, cover, reduce the heat to low, and simmer for about 1 hour, until the beef is very tender.

6. Stir in the navy beans and green beans, and cook for about 5 minutes, until heated through.

7. Remove the bay leaves, and season the stew with salt and freshly ground black pepper. Serve.

SUBSTITUTION TIP: If vegan or vegetarian stew better suits your needs, simply eliminate the beef, and replace the beef broth with vegetable broth. Reduce the cooking time to about 30 minutes, since the extra time is no longer required for the beef to cook in the broth.

PER SERVING Calories: 452; Carbs: 52g; Glycemic Load: 13; Fiber: 18g; Protein: 38g; Sodium: 246mg; Fat: 11g

10

ROAST BEEF with Wild Mushroom Sauce

PREP TIME: 20 MINUTES • COOK TIME: 50 MINUTES, PLUS 10 MINUTES STANDING TIME
SERVES 4

Roast beef graced many tables on Sunday evenings in days past, because this protein could cook while people attended church or enjoyed other activities. Grass-fed red meat is still an excellent option, since it contains conjugated linoleic acid (CLA), which can help correct impaired blood sugar metabolism.

2 teaspoons olive oil, plus extra for oiling the pan

Sea salt

Freshly ground black pepper

1 pound sirloin tip beef roast

8 ounces oyster mushrooms, sliced

4 ounces chanterelle mushrooms, sliced

4 ounces shiitake mushrooms, sliced

2 shallots, minced

1 teaspoon minced garlic

1 teaspoon chopped fresh thyme

3 tablespoons apple cider vinegar

½ cup coconut cream, skimmed off the top of canned coconut milk

1. Preheat the oven to 350°F.

2. Lightly oil a small roasting pan.

3. Lightly season the beef roast all over with salt and freshly ground black pepper, and place it in the roasting pan.

4. Roast for about 50 minutes for medium (internal temperature 155°F). Let the roast stand for 10 minutes before carving it

5. About 20 minutes before the end of the roasting time, make the sauce.

6. Put a large skillet over medium heat, and add the 2 teaspoons olive oil.

7. Sauté the mushrooms for about 10 minutes, until they start to caramelize.

8. Stir in the shallots, garlic, and thyme, and sauté for 3 minutes.

9. Stir in the apple cider vinegar and coconut cream. Sauté for about 5 minutes, until most of the liquid is absorbed.

10. Remove from heat and keep warm while you slice the roast.

11. Serve the beef with the wild mushroom sauce.

INGREDIENT TIP: Wild mushrooms are available dried if your local store does not have a nice selection of fresh ones. Plump up the dried mushrooms by soaking them in water for at least an hour before sautéing them for the sauce.

PER SERVING Calories: 414; Carbs: 11g; Glycemic Load: 2; Fiber: 3g; Protein: 35g; Sodium: 205mg; Fat: 14g

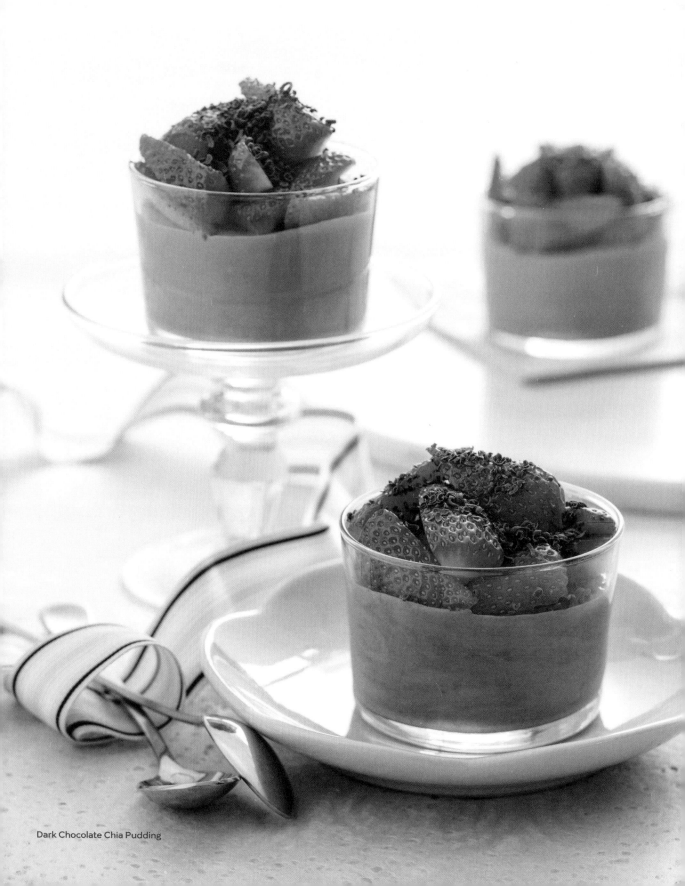

Dark Chocolate Chia Pudding

Drinks and Desserts

STRAWBERRY LEMONADE

PREP TIME: 5 MINUTES, PLUS 2 HOURS INFUSING TIME
SERVES 2

Lemonade can be stored in your refrigerator in a frosty pitcher for those times you need a thirst-quenching drink that isn't high in sugar. Fresh lemon and lime juice contain a great deal of pulp, so make sure you stir this beverage well. If you don't care for pulp, strain the lemonade first.

2 cups water

¾ cup freshly squeezed lemon juice

¼ cup freshly squeezed lime juice

1 tablespoon honey

1 cup sliced strawberries

4 ice cubes

1. In a medium nonreactive bowl, stir together the water, lemon juice, lime juice, and honey until well blended.

2. Stir in the strawberries, crushing them a little with the back of a spoon.

3. Put the bowl into the refrigerator for 2 hours to infuse the liquid.

4. Divide the ice cubes between 2 tall glasses.

5. Pour the strawberry lemonade into the glasses, and serve.

SUBSTITUTION TIP: Feel free to experiment with many different fruit and berries when creating this refreshing beverage. If a more intense flavor appeals to you, fresh peach or plum purée makes a superb addition, as well as freshly picked raspberries.

PER SERVING Calories :77; Carbs: 16g; Glycemic Load: 6; Fiber: 2g; Protein: 1g; Sodium: 19mg; Fat: 1g

ICED GREEN TEA WITH GINGER

PREP TIME: 10 MINUTES, PLUS 2 HOURS CHILLING TIME
SERVES 2

Iced tea is a tried and true method of quenching your thirst on a balmy day. Recall any movie you've seen about the Deep South: The heroines were always offering guests a frosted glass of this brew. Green tea is especially welcome because it is a powerful anti-inflammatory. Inflammation can impede the body's ability to absorb insulin, so anything that reduces inflammation helps manage blood sugar levels.

2 green tea bags

2-inch piece fresh ginger, peeled and grated

1 tablespoon chopped fresh mint

½ teaspoon chopped fresh thyme

3 cups boiling water

6 ice cubes

Fresh mint sprigs, for garnish

1. Put the tea bags, ginger, mint, and thyme in a medium bowl, and add the boiling water.

2. Stir and let the ingredients steep for 5 minutes.

3. Remove the tea bags, squeezing to remove all the liquid.

4. Pour the liquid through a fine-mesh sieve into a container, and discard the solids.

5. Chill the tea mixture completely in the refrigerator, about 2 hours.

6. Transfer the tea mixture to a blender, and add the ice cubes.

7. Process until the mixture is thick and smooth.

8. Serve the beverage garnished with mint sprigs.

SERVING TIP: You can also serve the green tea infusion straight over ice cubes without processing it in the blender. Add an extra cup of boiling water when preparing the tea to dilute the flavor a little if you are not blending the ice into the drink.

PER SERVING Calories: 11; Carbs: 2g; Glycemic Load: 0; Fiber: 0g; Protein: 0g; Sodium: 2mg; Fat: 0g

11

SPARKLING CANTALOUPE DRINK

PREP TIME: 15 MINUTES
SERVES 2

"Pale pastel" and "refreshing" are words you might use to describe this perfect summer beverage. Cantaloupe is packed with vitamins A and C, beta-carotene, and antioxidants. Look for melons that have a distinguishable sweet fragrance and feel heavy for their size.

2 cups diced cantaloupe

Juice of 2 limes

2 tablespoons chopped fresh mint

2 cups sparkling water

1. Put the cantaloupe, lime juice, and mint in a blender, and pulse until puréed.

2. Transfer the melon mixture to a measuring cup, and stir in the sparkling water.

3. Pour the beverage into 2 glasses, and serve.

SUBSTITUTION TIP: Honeydew melon and watermelon are other wonderful options for this refreshing beverage. The lime and mint work just as well with all melon choices.

PER SERVING Calories: 56; Carbs: 13g; Glycemic Load: 5; Fiber: 2g; Protein: 2g; Sodium: 29mg; Fat: 0g

11

GREEN PEAR PROTEIN SMOOTHIE

PREP TIME: 5 MINUTES
SERVES 2

Flaxseed isn't just packed with protein, it's also a wonderful source of omega-3 fatty acids, soluble fiber, and insoluble fiber. The fat and fiber are crucial for slowing digestion and reducing the speed at which sugar is absorbed. Add an extra teaspoon of flaxseed for a mega boost of these nutrients.

1 cup torn kale leaves

1 Bartlett pear, cored and chopped

½ English cucumber, cut into chunks

½ cup water

2 tablespoons sunflower seeds

1 teaspoon flaxseed

½ teaspoon ground nutmeg

4 ice cubes

1. Add the kale, pear, cucumber, water, sunflower seeds, flaxseed, and nutmeg to a blender.

2. Blend until the drink is smooth, and add the ice.

3. Blend with the ice until the drink is smooth and thick.

4. Pour the smoothie into 2 glasses, and serve.

INGREDIENT TIP: Sunflower seeds and flaxseed are packed with healthy protein, which makes this smoothie a stellar start to a busy day. Try to find roasted, unsalted sunflower seeds for optimum flavor.

PER SERVING Calories: 114; Carbs: 23g; Glycemic Load: 4; Fiber: 5g; Protein: 3g; Sodium: 18mg; Fat: 2g

11

FENNEL-CHARD SMOOTHIE

PREP TIME: 10 MINUTES
SERVES 2

Fennel often adds a huge burst of liquid when it is puréed, so try blending this smoothie first without adding water. Then add only enough so that the ingredients blend properly. Fennel is very high in antioxidants such as vitamin C, as well as fiber, folate, and potassium.

2 cups torn Swiss chard leaves

2 cups chopped fennel

1 peach, pitted and chopped

1 teaspoon orange zest

½ cup water

4 ice cubes

1. Put all the ingredients in a blender, and process until smooth.

2. Serve immediately.

INGREDIENT TIP: The subtle licorice flavor of the fennel plus the fresh orange zest create a smoothie that tastes exotic and fresh on the palate. Top each glass with feathery fennel fronds.

PER SERVING Calories: 53; Carbs: 12g; Glycemic Load: 6; Fiber: 2g; Protein: 4g; Sodium: 69mg; Fat: 0g

SUMMER VEGETABLE SMOOTHIE

PREP TIME: 15 MINUTES
SERVES 2

Starting your day with this smoothie gives you four servings of vegetables and one serving of fruit, a huge head-start on your daily requirements! Make sure you use a wooden spoon to stir your ingredients around a bit before blending. Otherwise the kale may sit on top without mixing in properly, since it is significantly lighter than the other fruits and vegetables.

2 celery stalks, chopped

1 apple, peeled, cored, and chopped

½ English cucumber, chopped

½ cup snap peas

2 cups shredded kale

Juice of ½ lemon

½ cup water

1 teaspoon grated fresh ginger

Pinch ground turmeric

1. Put all of the ingredients in a blender, and process until thick and smooth.

2. Add more water if you prefer a thinner beverage. Serve.

SERVING TIP: This recipe creates two generous portions that could be split into four smaller servings if you need to accommodate that number of people. The amount of nutritious vegetables in the smoothie ensures that you get at least half of your daily vegetable servings in one glass.

PER SERVING Calories: 124; Carbs: 28g; Glycemic Load: 5; Fiber: 6g; Protein: 5g; Sodium: 47mg; Fat: 0g

CREAMY GREEN APPLE SMOOTHIE

PREP TIME: 10 MINUTES
SERVES 2

You might think of fresh-cut grass when you sip this pastel smoothie for breakfast. It has an earthy herbal flavor with a touch of sweetness from the apple. If tart green types do not appeal to your taste, you can use a Red Delicious or Gala apple instead. This smoothie contains about one-third of your daily fiber requirement in one tasty glass.

2 cups spinach leaves

1 green apple, peeled, cored, and chopped

1 teaspoon chopped fresh thyme

1 cup unsweetened coconut milk (from a carton)

1 avocado, peeled and pitted

3 ice cubes

1. Blend the spinach, apple, thyme, coconut milk, and avocado together until smooth.

2. Add the ice cubes and blend until smooth and thick.

3. Serve immediately.

INGREDIENT TIP: This smoothie is very green and thick with a fresh flavor. If you're looking to add more fiber to your diet, simply don't peel the apple.

PER SERVING Calories: 286; Carbs: 23g; Glycemic Load: 3; Fiber: 10g; Protein: 3g; Sodium: 111mg; Fat: 22g

11

COCONUT MACAROONS

PREP TIME: 15 MINUTES, PLUS 1 HOUR CHILLING TIME • COOK TIME: 12 MINUTES

MAKES 12 COOKIES

A crispy melt-in-your-mouth cookie can finish off a lovely meal perfectly, especially with a steaming cup of herbal tea. These golden morsels do not have a high glycemic load; if you want a slightly sweeter cookie, add two more tablespoons of honey to the batter. This will bring the glycemic load up to 4 per cookie.

4 egg whites, at room temperature

Dash sea salt

1 teaspoon cream of tartar

2 tablespoons honey

2 teaspoons pure vanilla extract

2 cups unsweetened shredded coconut

Coconut oil, for greasing the baking sheet

INGREDIENT TIP: Egg whites at room temperature whip up higher and easier, so make sure you don't miss this step.

1. Put the egg whites in a large bowl with the salt, and beat them with an electric hand beater until foamy.

2. Add the cream of tartar, and beat the whites for about 4 minutes, until they form stiff peaks.

3. Carefully fold the honey, vanilla, and coconut into the egg whites.

4. Put the batter in the refrigerator for 1 hour to chill.

5. Preheat the oven to 350°F.

6. Line a baking sheet with parchment paper, and lightly grease it with coconut oil.

7. Drop the cookie batter onto the baking sheet by tablespoons.

8. Bake the cookies until the edges just start to brown, 8 to 12 minutes.

9. Cool the cookies on the baking sheet for 15 minutes, then remove them to wire racks to cool completely.

10. Store the cookies in a sealed container in the refrigerator for up to 1 week.

PER SERVING (1 cookie) Calories: 139; Carbs: 7g; Glycemic Load: 3; Fiber: 3g; Protein: 3g; Sodium: 38mg; Fat: 11g

CREAMY STRAWBERRY ICE CREAM

PREP TIME: 15 MINUTES, PLUS FREEZING TIME
MAKES 2 CUPS

You can create this luscious dessert without an ice cream maker by spreading the puréed and strained mixture into a metal baking dish, and placing the dish in the freezer. When it is frozen solid, pulse it in a processor until creamy. Serve the soft ice cream right away. Strawberries are satisfyingly sweet and packed with fiber, which can make you feel full longer.

2 cups sliced strawberries

1 avocado, peeled and pitted

½ cup unsweetened almond milk

1 teaspoon pure vanilla extract

1. Put the strawberries, avocado, almond milk, and vanilla in a food processor, and blend until puréed.

2. Pass the mixture through a fine-mesh sieve to catch all the strawberry seeds.

3. Put the strawberry mixture in an ice cream maker, and freeze according to the manufacturer's instructions.

SUBSTITUTION TIP: You can use rice milk in this recipe if you have a tree nut allergy. Rice milk has a lovely, fresh flavor and can be found in the dairy section of most grocery stores.

PER SERVING (½ cup) Calories: 134; Carbs: 10g; Glycemic Load: 2; Fiber: 5g; Protein: 2g; Sodium: 26mg; Fat: 11g

11

COCONUT CUSTARD

PREP TIME: 10 MINUTES • COOK TIME: 45 MINUTES

SERVES 4

Although there is no crunchy caramelized sugar on top, the touch of honey and smooth vanilla flavor in this custard will remind you of crème brûlée. Try adding a little pure almond extract, or a spoon of fresh blueberries as a garnish. Custards allow you to feel like you are cheating on your diet with an indulgent treat, when they are actually high in nutrients.

3 large eggs

1 tablespoon honey

2 teaspoons pure vanilla extract

¼ teaspoon ground nutmeg

Pinch sea salt

2 cups canned coconut milk

¼ cup unsweetened shredded coconut

COOKING TIP: The custard can also be made in 4 (6-ounce) ramekins for a more elegant presentation. The cooking time will be the same for the individual servings.

1. Preheat the oven to 350°F.

2. In a medium bowl, whisk together the eggs, honey, vanilla, nutmeg, and salt until blended.

3. Pour the coconut milk into a small saucepan, and put it on medium heat.

4. Bring the coconut milk to a simmer, remove it from the heat, and whisk it into the egg mixture.

5. Pass the mixture through a fine-mesh sieve into an 8-by-8-inch baking dish.

6. Place the baking dish in a larger baking dish, and pour hot water into the larger pan so that it comes about halfway up the custard pan, taking care not to spill any water into the mixture.

7. Bake the custard until a knife inserted in the center comes out clean, 45 to 50 minutes.

8. Let the custard pan cool on a wire rack for at least 1 hour.

9. Chill the custard in the refrigerator, and serve sprinkled with shredded coconut.

PER SERVING Calories: 146; Carbs: 7g; Glycemic Load: 3; Fiber: 1g; Protein: 6g; Sodium: 174mg; Fat: 10g

11

DARK CHOCOLATE CHIA PUDDING

PREP TIME: 15 MINUTES, PLUS 2 HOURS THICKENING TIME • COOK TIME: 5 MINUTES
SERVES 4

Sometimes chocolate is simply the only choice when it comes to dessert. The good news is that dark chocolate can help improve insulin sensitivity as well as reduce blood pressure and LDL cholesterol levels. However, chocolate should still be considered an indulgence, and limited to healthier recipes such as this rich pudding.

2 cups unsweetened almond milk

¼ cup unsweetened cocoa powder

2 tablespoons honey

1 teaspoon pure vanilla extract

½ cup chia seeds

Strawberries, for garnish (optional)

1. Put a small saucepan over low heat; add the almond milk, cocoa powder, honey, and vanilla, and stir to combine.

2. Heat for about 4 minutes, until the cocoa powder is completely dissolved.

3. Remove the liquid from the heat, and pour it into a medium bowl.

4. Stir in the chia seeds, and put the bowl in the refrigerator for about 2 hours, stirring every 30 minutes, until the pudding is thick.

5. Serve, garnished with fresh strawberries (if using).

COOKING TIP: Do not skimp on the soaking time, because the chia seeds need to soak up the liquid to get to their characteristic plumpness and produce the desired thick texture, like tapioca pudding. If you prefer a smoother texture, blend the pudding in a food processor or blender.

PER SERVING Calories: 125; Carbs: 19g; Glycemic Load: 5; Fiber: 7g; Protein: 5g; Sodium: 92mg; Fat: 8g

11

BUCKWHEAT CRÊPES with Berries

PREP TIME: 15 MINUTES • COOK TIME: 25 MINUTES
SERVES 4

Pancakes for dessert: What a concept! Crêpes are really just thin pancakes that can be wrapped around sweet or savory fillings. These crêpes get extra nutrition points for using buckwheat flour, packed with fiber, manganese, copper, and magnesium. Crêpes can be easily frozen between sheets of parchment paper. When thawing, they only need about 30 seconds in the microwave or 30 minutes defrosting at room temperature.

¾ cup buckwheat flour

¼ cup almond flour

¼ teaspoon ground nutmeg

Pinch sea salt

1 cup unsweetened almond milk, at room temperature

2 eggs, at room temperature

1 tablespoon melted coconut oil, plus more for cooking

2 cups mixed berries

SERVING TIP: Homemade applesauce, sliced peaches, fresh figs, and a smear of almond butter are all delectable choices for topping these crêpes if berries are not in season. You can eat them cold or warm.

1. In a medium bowl, stir together the buckwheat flour, almond flour, nutmeg, and salt.

2. In a small bowl, whisk together the almond milk, eggs, and coconut oil.

3. Stir the wet ingredients into the dry ingredients until the batter is well mixed.

4. Put a 9-inch skillet over medium heat, and brush it with coconut oil.

5. Add about ¼ cup batter to the skillet, and rotate the skillet so that the batter coats the bottom.

6. Cook the crêpe for about 2 minutes, until small bubbles appear on the surface, then flip it over.

7. Cook the second side of the crêpe for about 30 seconds, and remove it from the skillet to a plate.

8. Repeat with the remaining batter until there are 8 crêpes total.

9. Divide the berries evenly between the crêpes, rolling them up around the fruit and serving 2 per person.

PER SERVING Calories: 181; Carbs: 23g; Glycemic Load: 14; Fiber: 4g; Protein: 7g; Sodium: 138mg; Fat: 8g

11

BROWN RICE PUDDING

PREP TIME: 5 MINUTES • COOK TIME: 30 MINUTES
SERVES 4

Rice pudding is a popular dish, seen at backroad diners and four-star restaurants alike. This version falls somewhere in between, with fiber-rich pear, warm spices, and a crunchy topping of healthy almonds. Curl up with a warm bowl of rice pudding in your favorite comfy chair when you need to unwind and decompress from the day.

2 cups unsweetened almond milk

1 cup brown rice

1 pear, peeled, cored, and grated

1 teaspoon pure vanilla extract

½ teaspoon ground cinnamon

Pinch ground cloves

Pinch ground nutmeg

Pinch sea salt

2 tablespoons slivered almonds

1. In a large saucepan, stir together the almond milk, rice, pear, vanilla, cinnamon, cloves, nutmeg, and salt.

2. Put the saucepan over medium heat, and bring the mixture to a simmer.

3. Reduce the heat to low and simmer, stirring frequently, for about 30 minutes, until the rice is tender and most of the liquid is absorbed.

4. Serve the pudding topped with almonds.

COOKING TIP: You might have to add a little extra almond milk while cooking this dessert if you like your pudding a bit thinner in texture. The pudding will thicken as it cools, so you can also wait until you are ready to serve it to adjust the consistency.

PER SERVING Calories: 191; Carbs: 35g; Glycemic Load: 18; Fiber: 3g; Protein: 4g; Sodium: 151mg; Fat: 4g

APPLE-ALMOND CRUMBLE

PREP TIME: 20 MINUTES · COOK TIME: 30 MINUTES

SERVES 6

If you are craving a treat that reminds you of home, this apple crumble should fill the bill. The scent of spiced apples and toasting oats will waft through your kitchen as it bakes. Try it with a scoop of coconut milk ice cream, either homemade or a limited-ingredient product from your grocery store.

FOR THE TOPPING

1 cup rolled oats

½ cup ground almonds

1 tablespoon honey

3 tablespoons coconut oil

FOR THE FILLING

2 teaspoons coconut oil

8 apples, peeled, cored, and thinly sliced

1 teaspoon ground cinnamon

¼ teaspoon ground nutmeg

Pinch ground cloves

INGREDIENT TIP: If gluten is an issue in your diet, take a look at the label on the oats you purchase to ensure they are manufactured in a gluten-free facility. Oats are gluten-free, but cross-contamination with gluten-containing products can often be an issue.

TO MAKE THE TOPPING

1. In a small bowl, stir together the oats, ground almonds, and honey.

2. Add the coconut oil, and use your fingertips to rub it into the oat mixture until the topping resembles coarse crumbs.

TO MAKE THE FILLING

1. Preheat the oven to 375°F.

2. Put a large skillet on medium heat, and add the coconut oil.

3. Sauté the apple slices for about 5 minutes, until they are tender-crisp.

4. Stir the cinnamon, nutmeg, and cloves into the apples, and transfer the mixture to a 9-by-13-inch baking dish.

5. Spread the filling out in the dish, and top the fruit evenly with the topping mixture.

6. Bake for about 25 minutes, until the apples are bubbly and the topping is golden brown.

7. Serve warm.

PER SERVING Calories: 308; Carbs: 48g; Glycemic Load: 13; Fiber: 9g; Protein: 4g; Sodium: 3mg; Fat: 14g

MOIST CARROT CAKE

PREP TIME: 20 MINUTES • COOK TIME: 45 MINUTES
SERVES 8

You can create your own chia seed flour by tossing chia seeds in your food processor and pulsing until they are very finely ground. The benefits are worth noting: Chia seeds have been linked to a reduction of insulin resistance contributing to belly fat, and are very high in fiber and omega-3 fatty acids, both of which lower blood sugar levels in the body.

¼ cup melted coconut oil, plus more for greasing the pan

½ cup chia seed flour, plus extra for dusting the pans

2½ cups almond flour

2 teaspoons ground cinnamon

1 teaspoon baking soda

½ teaspoon ground nutmeg

¼ teaspoon ground ginger

¼ teaspoon sea salt

Pinch ground cloves

5 large eggs

¼ cup honey

2 teaspoons pure vanilla extract

3 cups finely shredded carrots

½ cup chopped pecans

11

1. Preheat the oven to 325°F.

2. Lightly grease a 9-by-13-inch baking dish, and dust it with chia seed flour. Set aside.

3. In a large bowl, stir together the chia seed flour, almond flour, cinnamon, baking soda, nutmeg, ginger, salt, and cloves.

4. In a medium bowl, whisk together the eggs, honey, ¼ cup coconut oil, and vanilla.

5. Add the wet ingredients to the dry, and stir to combine.

6. Stir in the carrots and pecans until the batter is well blended.

7. Transfer the batter to the baking pan, and tap it on the counter to remove any bubbles.

8. Bake the cake until a knife inserted in the middle comes out clean, 40 to 45 minutes.

9. Remove the cake from the oven, and cool it on a wire rack.

10. Chill the cake in the refrigerator, covered in plastic wrap, until you are ready to serve it.

COOKING TIP: If you want to create a layer cake instead of a sheet cake, use 2 (6-inch) round cake pans instead of the baking dish. Frost your cake with cinnamon-spiked whipped coconut cream, and serve.

PER SERVING Calories: 249; Carbs: 18g; Glycemic Load: 10; Fiber: 3g; Protein: 9g; Sodium: 293mg; Fat: 17g

11

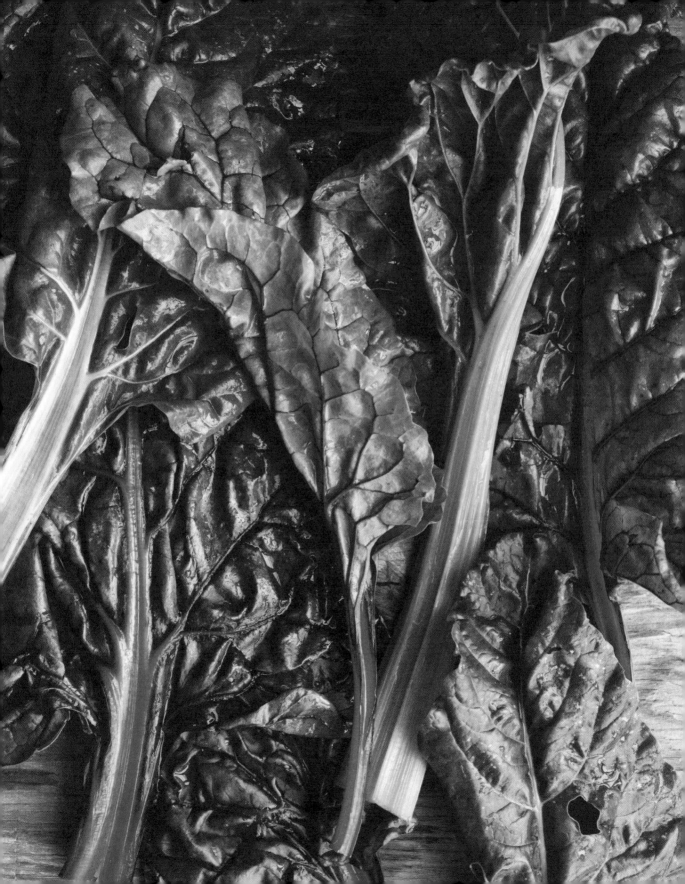

RESOURCES

The following list of additional resources provides more information about insulin resistance and its associated conditions, self-compassion, and positive body image.

› **The American Diabetes Association** website contains useful information about recognizing, living with, and managing type 2 diabetes. It is a national organization for health professionals and consumers, and almost every state has a local office.
www.diabetes.org

› **Beauty Redefined** is a website run by a pair of twins who have PhDs in the study of media and body image. Their aim is to challenge the norms of beauty in the media, and change people's perceptions of their bodies from the inside out.
www.beautyredefined.net

› **The Center for Young Women's Health** is targeted to younger women who struggle with their self-esteem and body image. The website also contains helpful information about PCOS.
www.youngwomenshealth.org/2012/05/30/self-esteem

› **The National Diabetes Education Program** is sponsored by the US National Institutes of Health and the US Centers for Disease Control and Prevention. The federally funded program aims to improve diabetes treatment methods, promote early diagnosis, and prevent or delay the development of diabetes.
www.ndep.nih.gov

› **The National Eating Disorders Association** is a nonprofit organization for those affected by eating disorders. Having poor body image is an early trigger for developing an eating disorder, and this website contains a number of articles to help one construct a positive body image.
www.nationaleatingdisorders.org
/developing-and-maintaining-positive-body-image

> **The National Institute of Diabetes and Digestive and Kidney Diseases** website provides full scientific breakdowns of the development of insulin resistance and prediabetes, for those who seek a better understanding of their condition.
www.niddk.nih.gov/health-information/health-topics/Diabetes/insulin-resistance-prediabetes

> **The PCOS Awareness Association** is a nonprofit organization that aims to spread awareness about PCOS. The founders of the website hope to increase early diagnosis rates and overcome the various individual symptoms of the condition.
www.pcosaa.org

> **Self-Compassion**, Dr. Kristen Neff's website, contains more information about the subject matter discussed in chapter 2, and includes helpful written, spoken, and meditative exercises to help you practice self-compassion.
www.self-compassion.org

REFERENCES

Alberti, K., R. Eckel, S. Grundy, P. Zimmet, J. Cleeman, K. Donato, J. Fruchart, W. James, C. Loria, and S. Smith. "Harmonizing the Metabolic Syndrome: A Joint Interim Statement of the International Diabetes Federation Task Force on Epidemiology and Prevention; National Heart, Lung, and Blood Institute; American Heart Association; World Heart Federation; International Atherosclerosis Society; and International Association for the Study of Obesity." *Circulation* 120, no. 1 (October 2009): 1640–45 . doi:10.1161/CIRCULATIONAHA.109.192644.

American Heart Association. "Managing Blood Pressure with a Heart-Healthy Diet." Last updated October 23, 2015. www.heart.org/HEARTORG/Conditions /HighBloodPressure/PreventionTreatmentofHighBloodPressure/Managing-Blood-Pressure-with-a-Heart-Healthy-Diet_UCM_301879_Article.jsp#.

Biaggioni, I., and S. Davis. "Caffeine: A Cause of Insulin Resistance?" *Diabetes Care* 25, no. 2 (February 2002): 399–400.

Centers for Disease Control and Prevention. "2014 National Diabetes Statistics Report." Last updated May 15, 2015. www.cdc.gov/diabetes/data/statistics /2014statisticsreport.html.

Colberg, S., R. Sigal, B. Fernhall, J. Regensteiner, B. Blissmer, R. Rubin, L. Chasan-Taber, A. Allbright, and B. Braun. "Exercise and Type 2 Diabetes." *Diabetes Care* 33, no. 12 (December 2010): 147–67.

Diabetic Care Services. "What You Need to Know about Insulin Resistance and Pre-Diabetes." Accessed November 22, 2015. www.diabeticcareservices.com/diabetes-education /prediabetes-and-insulin-resistance.

Dunaif, A. "Insulin Resistance and the Polycystic Ovary Syndrome: Mechanism and Implications for Pathogenesis." *Endocrine Reviews* 18, no. 6 (1997): 774–800.

Gunnars, K. "6 Reasons Why a Calorie Is Not a Calorie." *Authority Nutrition.* November 2015. authoritynutrition.com/6-reasons-why-a-calorie-is-not-a-calorie.

Healthy Women. "Polycystic Ovary Syndrome." Last updated December 2, 2015. www.healthywomen.org/condition/polycystic-ovary-syndrome.

Helmrich, S., D. Ragland, R. Leung, and R. Paffenbarger. "Physical Activity and Reduced Occurrence of Non-Insulin-Dependent Diabetes Mellitus." *New England Journal of Medicine* 325, no. 3 (1991): 147–52. doi:10.1056/NEJM199107183250302.

Hignett, W., and T. Kyle. "Polycystic Ovarian Syndrome (PCOS) and Obesity." *Your Weight Matters Magazine.* Spring 2011. www.obesityaction.org/educational-resources /resource-articles-2/obesity-related-diseases/polycystic-ovarian-syndrome-pcos- and-obesity.

Hutchison, P. "How Many Calories a Day Does the Average Body Burn?" *Livestrong.* February 7, 2014. www.livestrong.com/article/315121-how-many-calories-a-day-does- the-average-body-burn.

Jornayvaz, F., M. Jurczak, H. Lee, A. Birkenfeld, D. Frederick, D. Zhang, X. Zhang, V. Samuel, and G. Shulman. "A High-Fat, Ketogenic Diet Causes Hepatic Insulin Resis- tance in Mice, Despite Increasing Energy Expenditure and Preventing Weight Gain." *American Journal of Physiology Endocrinology and Metabolism* 299, no. 5 (November 2010): 805–15. doi:10.1152/ajpendo.00361.2010.

Knowler, W., E. Barrett-Connor, S. Fowler, R. Hamman, J. Lachin, E. Walker, and D. Nathan. "Reduction in the Incidence of Type 2 Diabetes with Lifestyle Intervention or Metformin." *New England Journal of Medicine (Diabetes Prevention Program Research Group)* 346, no. 6 (February 2002): 393–403.

Kraegen, E., P. Clark, A. Jenkins, E. Daley, D. Chisholm, and L. Storlien. "Development of Muscle Insulin Resistance After Liver Insulin Resistance in High-Fat-Fed Rats." *Diabetes* 40, no. 11 (November 1991): 1397–1403.

Lee, M., and K. Fujioka. "Dietary Prescriptions for the Overweight Patient: The Poten- tial Benefits of Low-Carbohydrate Diets in Insulin Resistance." *Diabetes, Obesity and Metabolism* 13, no. 3 (March 2011): 204–6.

Livingstone, C., and M. Collinson. "Sex Steroids and Insulin Resistance." *Clinical Science* 102, no. 2 (February 2002): 151–56.

Mayo Clinic. "Dietary Fats: Know Which Types to Choose." August 7, 2014. www.mayoclinic .org/healthy-lifestyle/nutrition-and-healthy-eating/in-depth/fat/art-20045550.

Mayo Clinic. "Metabolism and Weight Loss: How You Burn Calories." September 19, 2014. www.mayoclinic.org/healthy-lifestyle/weight-loss/in-depth/metabolism /art-20046508.

McMillan-Price, J., and J. Brand-Miller. "Low-Glycaemic Index Diets and Body Weight Regulation." *International Journal of Obesity* 30, no. 1 (2006): 40–46. doi:10.1038 /sj.ijo.0803491.

Nassis, G., K. Papantakou, K. Skenderi, M. Triandafillopoulou, S. Kavouras, M. Yannakoulia, G. Chrousos, and L. Sidossis. "Aerobic Exercise Training Improves Insulin Sensitivity without Changes in Body Weight, Body Fat, Adiponectin, and Inflammatory Markets in Overweight and Obese Girls." *Metabolism* 54, no. 11 (November 2005): 1472–79.

National Institute of Diabetes and Digestive and Kidney Diseases. "Insulin Resistance and Prediabetes." June 2014. www.niddk.nih.gov/health-information/health-topics /Diabetes/insulin-resistance-prediabetes/Pages/index.aspx.

Nelson, R., J. Horowitz, R. Holleman, A. Swartz, S. Strath, A. Kriska, and C. Richardson. "Daily Physical Activity Predicts Degree of Insulin Resistance: A Cross-Sectional Observational Study Using the 2003–2004 National Health and Nutrition Examination Survey." *International Journal of Behavioral Nutrition and Physical Activity* 10, no. 10 (January 2013). doi:10.1186/1479-5868-10-10.

O'Meara., A. "The Percentage of People Who Regain Weight after Rapid Weight Loss and the Risks of Doing So." February 18, 2015. www.livestrong.com/article/438395 -the-percentage-of-people-who-regain-weight-after-rapid-weight-loss-risks.

Prevention. "10 Diet Mistakes Seriously Slowing Your Metabolism." December 16, 2014. www.prevention.com/weight-loss/weight-loss-tips/common-diet-mistakes-slow -metabolism.

Sanchez-Villegas, A., and M. Martinez-Gonzalez. "Diet, a New Target to Prevent Depression?" *BMC Medicine* 11, no. 3 (January 2013). doi:10.1186/1741-7015-11-3.

Targher, G., M. Alberiche, M. Zenere, R. Bonadonna, M. Muggeo, and E. Bonora. "Cigarette Smoking and Insulin Resistance in Patients with Noninsulin-dependent Diabetes Mellitus." *Journal of Clinical Endocrinology and Metabolism* 82, no. 11 (1997): 3619–24.

Trumbo, P., S. Schlicker, A. Yates, and M. Poos. "Dietary Reference Intakes for Energy, Carbohydrate, Fiber, Fat, Fatty Acids, Cholesterol, Protein, and Amino Acids." *Journal of the American Dietetic Association* 102, no. 11 (2002): 1621–30.

Tylka, T. "Development and Psychometric Evaluation of a Measure of Intuitive Eating." *Journal of Counseling Psychology* 53, no. 2 (April 2006): 226-240.

Van Der Heijden, G., Z. Wang, Z. Chu, G. Toffolo, E. Manesso, P. Sauer, and A. Sunehag. "Strength Exercise Improves Muscle Mass and Hepatic Insulin Sensitivity in Obese Youth." *Medicine & Science in Sports & Exercise* 42, no. 11 (November 2010): 1973–80. doi:10.1249/MSS.0b013e3181df16d9.

Yajnik, C., C. Joglekar, A. Pandit, A. Bavdekar, S. Bapat, S. Bhave, S. Leary, and C. Fall. "Higher Offspring Birth Weight Predicts the Metabolic Syndrome in Mothers but Not Fathers 8 Years after Delivery." *Diabetes* 52, no. 8 (August 2003): 2090–96.

You and Your Hormones. "Insulin." Accessed November 19, 2015. www.yourhormones.info/hormones/insulin.aspx.

GLYCEMIC INDEX AND GLYCEMIC LOAD FOOD LISTS

The following is a list of the glycemic index and glycemic load of many common carbohydrates. Foods are ranked between 0 and 100 based on how they affect one's blood glucose level. The best choices are low glycemic, which have a rating of 55 or less, and medium glycemic, which have a rating of 56 to 69.

Remember that it is more important to pay attention to the glycemic load of a food, that is, the amount of carbohydrates it contains per serving. The best choices have low (less than 10) or moderate (between 10 and 20) loads.

GLYCEMIC INDEX AND GLYCEMIC LOAD OF COMMON FOODS

FOOD	GLYCEMIC INDEX	SERVING SIZE (GRAMS)	GLYCEMIC LOAD (PER SERVING)
BAKERY PRODUCTS			
Bagel, white	72	70	25
Baguette, white	95	30	15
Barley bread	34	30	7
Corn tortilla	52	50	12
Croissant	67	57	17
Doughnut	76	47	17
Pita bread	68	30	10
Sourdough rye	48	30	6
Soya and linseed bread	36	30	3
Sponge cake	46	63	17

FOOD	GLYCEMIC INDEX	SERVING SIZE (GRAMS)	GLYCEMIC LOAD (PER SERVING)
Wheat tortilla	30	50	8
White wheat flour bread	71	30	10
Whole-wheat bread	71	30	9
BEVERAGES			
Apple juice, unsweetened	44	250mL	30
Coca-Cola	63	250mL	16
Gatorade	78	250mL	12
Lucozade	95	250mL	40
Orange juice, unsweetened	50	250mL	12
Tomato juice, canned	38	250mL	4
BREAKFAST CEREALS			
All-Bran	55	30	12
Coco Pops	77	30	20
Cornflakes	93	30	23
Muesli	66	30	16
Oatmeal	55	50	13
Special K	69	30	14
DAIRY			
Ice cream, regular	57	50	6
Milk, full fat	41	250mL	5
Milk, skim	32	250mL	4
Reduced-fat yogurt with fruit	33	200	11
FRUITS			
Apple	39	120	6
Banana, ripe	62	120	16
Cherries	22	120	3
Dates, dried	42	60	18
Grapefruit	25	120	3
Grapes	59	120	11
Mango	41	120	8
Orange	40	120	4
Peach	42	120	5
Pear	38	120	4
Pineapple	51	120	8
Raisins	64	60	28

FOOD	GLYCEMIC INDEX	SERVING SIZE (GRAMS)	GLYCEMIC LOAD (PER SERVING)
Strawberries	40	120	1
Watermelon	72	120	4
GRAINS			
Brown rice	50	150	16
Buckwheat	45	150	13
Bulgur	30	50	11
Corn on the cob	60	150	20
Couscous	65	150	9
Fettucini	32	180	15
Gnocchi	68	180	33
Macaroni	47	180	23
Quinoa	53	150	13
Spaghetti, white	46	180	22
Spaghetti, whole-wheat	42	180	26
Vermicelli	35	180	16
White rice	89	150	43
LEGUMES			
Baked beans	40	150	6
Black beans	30	150	7
Butter beans	36	150	8
Chickpeas	10	150	3
Kidney beans	29	150	7
Lentils	29	150	5
Navy beans	31	150	9
Soybeans	50	150	1
SNACK FOODS			
Cashews, salted	27	50	3
Corn chips, salted	42	50	11
Fruit Roll-Ups	99	30	24
Graham crackers	74	25	14
Honey	61	25	12
Hummus	6	30	0
M&M's, peanut	33	30	6
Microwave popcorn, plain	55	20	6
Muesli bar	61	30	13
Nutella	33	20	4

FOOD	GLYCEMIC INDEX	SERVING SIZE (GRAMS)	GLYCEMIC LOAD (PER SERVING)
Peanuts	7	50	0
Potato chips	51	50	12
Pretzels	83	30	16
Rice cakes	82	25	17
Rye crisps	64	25	11
Shortbread	64	25	10
Vanilla wafers	77	25	14
VEGETABLES			
Beetroot	64	80	4
Carrot	35	80	2
Green peas	51	80	4
Parsnip	52	80	4
Sweet potato	70	150	22
White potato, boiled	81	150	22
Yam	54	150	20

Sources: Harvard Health Publications (http://www.health.harvard.edu/healthy-eating/glycemic_index_and_glycemic_load_for_100_foods) and Mendosa.com (http://www.mendosa.com/gilists.htm).

CONVERSION TABLES

VOLUME EQUIVALENTS (LIQUID)

US STANDARD	US STANDARD (OUNCES)	METRIC (APPROXIMATE)
2 tablespoons	1 fl. oz.	30 mL
¼ cup	2 fl. oz.	60 mL
½ cup	4 fl. oz.	120 mL
1 cup	8 fl. oz.	240 mL
1½ cups	12 fl. oz.	355 mL
2 cups or 1 pint	16 fl. oz.	475 mL
4 cups or 1 quart	32 fl. oz.	1 L
1 gallon	128 fl. oz.	4 L

OVEN TEMPERATURES

FAHRENHEIT (F)	CELSIUS (C) (APPROXIMATE)
250°F	120°C
300°F	150°C
325°F	165°C
350°F	180°C
375°F	190°C
400°F	200°C
425°F	220°C
450°F	230°C

VOLUME EQUIVALENTS (DRY)

US STANDARD	METRIC (APPROXIMATE)
⅛ teaspoon	0.5 mL
¼ teaspoon	1 mL
½ teaspoon	2 mL
¾ teaspoon	4 mL
1 teaspoon	5 mL
1 tablespoon	15 mL
¼ cup	59 mL
⅓ cup	79 mL
½ cup	118 mL
⅔ cup	156 mL
¾ cup	177 mL
1 cup	235 mL
2 cups or 1 pint	475 mL
3 cups	700 mL
4 cups or 1 quart	1 L

WEIGHT EQUIVALENTS

US STANDARD	METRIC (APPROXIMATE)
½ ounce	15 g
1 ounce	30 g
2 ounces	60 g
4 ounces	115 g
8 ounces	225 g
12 ounces	340 g
16 ounces or 1 pound	455 g

THE DIRTY DOZEN AND CLEAN FIFTEEN

A nonprofit and environmental watchdog organization called Environmental Working Group (EWG) looks at data supplied by the US Department of Agriculture (USDA) and the Food and Drug Administration (FDA) about pesticide residues. Each year it compiles a list of the best and worst pesticide loads found in commercial crops. You can use these lists to decide which fruits and vegetables to buy organic to minimize your exposure to pesticides and which produce is considered safe enough to buy conventionally. This does not mean they are pesticide-free, though, so wash these fruits and vegetables thoroughly.

These lists change every year, so make sure you look up the most recent one before you fill your shopping cart. You'll find the most recent lists as well as a guide to pesticides in produce at EWG.org/FoodNews.

2015 DIRTY DOZEN

Apples
Celery
Cherry tomatoes
Cucumbers
Grapes
Nectarines (imported)
Peaches
Potatoes
Snap peas (imported)
Spinach
Strawberries
Sweet bell peppers

In addition to the Dirty Dozen, the EWG added two types of produce contaminated with highly toxic organo-phosphate insecticides:

Kale/collard greens
Hot peppers

2015 CLEAN FIFTEEN

Asparagus
Avocados
Cabbage
Cantaloupes (domestic)
Cauliflower
Eggplants
Grapefruits
Kiwis

Mangos
Onions
Papayas
Pineapples
Sweet corn
Sweet peas (frozen)
Sweet potatoes

RECIPE INDEX

INDEX